What Athletes and Teachers Have to Say About *Eating for Endurance*

"*Eating for Endurance* is a very readable primer on nutrition in general and sports nutrition in particular. There is a wealth of basic information here, placed in a practical context . . . this is a job well done."

— *David L. Costill*
Director, Human Performance Laboratory
Ball State University

"*Eating for Endurance* will have a strong appeal to endurance athletes like myself, but will be valuable to all people who realize that their on-going health/fitness is up to them. Nutrition used to be overwhelmed by misinformation — the publication of this book indicates how far sports medicine has come in this area. The information in the book is crucial to athletes today."

— *Bill Rodgers*
Four-time winner of the Boston Marathon
and four-time winner of the New York Marathon

"The best book ever written on the subject. After reading Coleman's *Eating for Endurance*, I changed my diet, won the Western States 100 mile run, and thanked her for improving my times."

— *Sally Edwards*
Author of *The Triathlon Training and Fitness Book*

"I am very impressed with this published edition of *Eating for Endurance*. I have used the book before as an optional text, but it is so valuable that now I am going to require it. The charts, diet tips, and menus are excellent for the students."

— *Barbara Wright, M.A.*
Professor of Physical Education
Orange Coast College
Costa Mesa, California

"There are three major physical variables in endurance — genetics, training, and nutrition. Nothing can be done about the first. Everything has been written about the second. The third, nutrition, is perhaps the most important and least understood of all. There are no "quick fixes" in sports, but if there is anything that can be changed quickly to produce dramatic results, it's your nutrition. Coleman's book is well researched, scientifically and personally — as Ellen is not only a scholar, but an athlete. I give this book my highest recommendation."

— *Michael Shermer*
Ultra-Marathon Cyclist and
Co-founder of the Race Across America

"*Eating for Endurance* is excellent. Using charts effectively to summarize and explain concepts, it covers its subject comprehensively and in an easy-to-understand way. I plan to use it as a required text both at San Diego State University and Mesa College."

— *Christine DuPraw, R.D., M.P.H.*
Professor of Sports Nutrition

"*Eating for Endurance* is really informative. It uses a lot of examples, showing actual comparisons of athletes while they are competing, and what happens to them nutritionally. Ellen Coleman covers every topic for the athlete — carbohydrates, carbohydrate-loading, fats, caffeine, the whole works. She doesn't overlook anything. Overall I think it is an excellent book."

— *Dave Scott*
Six-time Ironman Triathlon Champion
Author of *Dave Scott's Triathlon Training*

Eating for Endurance

Revised Edition

Ellen Coleman, R.D., M.A., M.P.H.

Bull Publishing Company

PALO ALTO, CALIFORNIA

ISBN 0-923521-13-5
Printed in the United States
All rights reserved

Bull Publishing Company
P.O. Box 208
Palo Alto, California 94302
(415) 322-2855

Distributed in the United States by:
Publishers Group West
4065 Hollis Street
Emeryville, California 94608

Library of Congress Cataloging-in-Publication Data

Coleman, Ellen.
    Eating for endurance / Ellen Coleman. — ed.
        p.   cm.
    Includes bibliographical references and index.
    ISBN 0-923521-13-5 : $12.95
    1. Athletes—Nutrition. 2. Nutrition. 3.Exercise—Physiological
aspects. 4. Energy metabolism.   I. Title.
RC1235.C63   1992
613.2'024796—dc20   91-39344
                                                                CIP

Cover Design: Robb Pawlak
Cover Photo: Steven Oto
Athlete on cover: Barbara Martinelli
Interior Design: Maura McAndrew
Production Manager: Helen O'Donnell
Compositior: Shadow Canyon Graphics
Printer: Bookcrafters, Inc.

Contents

Preface

After running the first 23 miles of a marathon at a fast sub 6-minutes-per-mile pace, the lead runner's legs suddenly stiffen up and she can barely run the last few miles at a much slower 8-minute pace. Several runners pass her before she reaches the finish line because her leg muscles have run out of their stored sugar supply.

In the third hour of a four-hour bicycle race, the lead rider falls off his bike and starts to convulse. He has lost the race because he bonked. His liver has run out of its stored sugar supply and his blood sugar has dropped to dangerously-low levels.

With the score tied and 3 seconds to go in the game, the quarterback attempts to throw a long pass. His intended receiver, the tight end, is behind the last defensive back, but the pass falls short. His arm muscles have lost accuracy and strength because they have used up much of their stored sugar supply.

All of these athletes could have improved their performances by following sound scientific principles of sports nutrition. Twenty-five years ago, it was common for athletes to eat high-protein diets, to reduce their intake of food on the days before competition, to skip breakfast or eat steak on the day of competition, to take no refreshment or liquids during competition, and to eat very little after competition. At present, knowledgeable athletes follow none of these old regimens.

Sports nutrition is so scientific that any athlete who does not follow the basic rules of eating for competing will be at a marked disadvantage to those who know how to eat properly.

Not only are good eating habits necessary for successful competition in sports, they are also necessary for optimum health. Fifty percent of the death certificates in the United States today cite heart attacks as the cause of death. Most of these deaths could have been prevented or, at least, been delayed by proper nutrition. Obesity predisposes people to heart attacks, strokes, high blood pressure, gallstones and cancer of the uterus, breast, prostate and colon. Proper exercise and eating habits can help to prevent and treat obesity.

How, what and when you eat is important to both your ability to compete in sports and your ability to avoid certain diseases. This book will help you to eat for sport and health. I hope you will read and follow the scientific principles that are outlined.

Gabe Mirkin, M.D.
11/9/87

Table of Figures

Chapter 1

Oxygen is Everything

How Oxygen Use Affects Performance

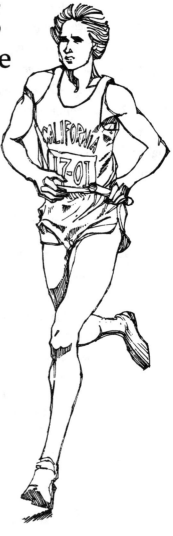

You get out with the front runners, breathing hard. You know that you're pushing it, but feel good.

You pass the second mile, still feeling good. You feel proud. You're flying.

At the third mile you know you're on the way to a record time. You never trained at a pace this fast. It hurts but you're cruising.

By the fourth mile, though, your running style becomes less fluid. You struggle with the pace. Your legs feel heavy. You have to cut back.

When you pass the fifth mile, you're back in control. Your time at the finish is slow, two minutes slower than your average.

It may have been the first time you went out front. You stayed ahead of the pack for the first half of the race, and paid for it in the second half. You could have possibly run the same time, or a faster time with less pain if you had paced yourself more evenly.

"But I had a record time at the three mile mark!" you exclaim. "What happened?"

Your body's ability to use oxygen determines in large part your endurance capacity. There are two interrelated energy systems, one dependent on oxygen and the other able to function without oxygen — but the one that doesn't use oxygen is severely limited, and can easily be exhausted. It is important to understand in a general way how this works, because it explains why what you eat and how you train can make all the difference in how you perform in an endurance event.

In this chapter the two energy systems are described, along with their general relationship to the sources of energy in the food we eat.

Metabolism and the Energy Pathways

Our bodies run on food, water and oxygen. We all know that we need these vital substances, but most of us don't know how their use is interrelated. Most of our ideas (and myths) about sources of energy relate to food. There are plenty of theories in fashion — ask any health food store clerk. Most don't have much to do with how our bodies function, and most people don't spend much time wondering about the connections between food and human performance. It relates in very important ways to our use of oxygen.

As I said above, there are two related energy systems: one that requires no oxygen, and is called *anaerobic*, and one that is dependent on a ready supply of oxygen, and is called *aerobic*.

Chains of chemical reactions utilize food and oxygen

(and water) to make the body go. This is referred to as *metabolism*. Anaerobic metabolism is the series of reactions, requiring no oxygen, which provides immediate energy. It soon needs help, however, from the oxygen-dependent aerobic energy system.

At home or work, your body is probably idling. You can get by with a minimum amount of food (or calories) and oxygen. When you begin to exercise, however, the demand for energy increases and so the demand for oxygen increases. When the exercise lasts beyond several minutes, the body needs a continuous supply of oxygen, as it starts depending on aerobic metabolism.

The chemical processes that produce energy take place in the individual cells of your muscles. For a brief period of time, less than two minutes, your body can work at a rate which exceeds your ability to make oxygen available to your muscles, depending almost entirely on anaerobic metabolism.

For a limited time, this is a very effective source. Anaerobic metabolism is one of our built-in survival mechanisms: It protects us at moments when we can't supply oxygen fast enough, for instance when we have a sudden need either to fight or flee from danger.

The interplay between aerobic and anaerobic metabolism is one of the most fascinating and challenging aspects of human performance. Neither the aerobic nor the anaerobic metabolic pathway works exclusively to supply energy during exercise. They work together, each complementing and supporting the other, as length and type of exercise affect demands for and sources of energy.

Understanding how the aerobic and anaerobic pathways work together to supply energy will help you understand which fuel the muscles use during a given exercise. It will help you appreciate the relationship between food as a part of your diet and food as your fuel for performance. It will also help you choose the right foods, and learn to train and finally to pace yourself for optimum performance. Training prepares your body, and affects your body's capacity to supply and utilize oxygen. Pacing affects the order in which available energy sources are used. So all three — eating, training, and pacing — interact to have a very important effect on how well you perform.

The Energy Sources

An energy-rich compound called adenosine triphosphate (ATP) is used for all energy-requiring processes within your cells. The muscle cell produces and maintains ongoing supplies of ATP, utilizing glucose from carbohydrates, fatty acids from fats, and to some extent amino acids from proteins.

Glucose

Glucose comes from food high in carbohydrate, such as fruits, vegetables, breads, cereals, grains, pasta, beans and sweets. Glucose is stored in muscles and the liver as a substance called *glycogen*, which is actually a long chain of glucose molecules hooked together.

Although food eaten before and even during exercise can supply some carbohydrate for energy through your bloodstream, the main carbohydrate energy source is the glycogen you have stored ahead of time. For 30-60 minutes it will be almost your only energy source, and after 90 minutes your performance may begin to deteriorate as your glycogen stores are depleted. Training and diet affect how much you can store. Training and pacing determine how rapidly it is used up during exercise.

There is a two-stage chemical process to break down glucose for energy. (See Figure 1)

Figure 1
The Two Energy Systems

Only carbohydrates, in the form of glucose, can be utilized anaerobically, without oxygen. The process is inefficient, extracting only a small part of the energy potentially available from the glucose; but it is also rapid, and thus furnishes the energy for short-term bursts of exercise.

If oxygen is available, the product of the anaerobic reaction is then utilized aerobically, utilizing the full energy potential (18 or 19 times as much). The aerobic process can also utilize fats (and even proteins), which, unlike carbohydrates, are available in the body in virtually unlimited amounts. Thus the availability of oxygen in large part determines the potential for endurance exercise.

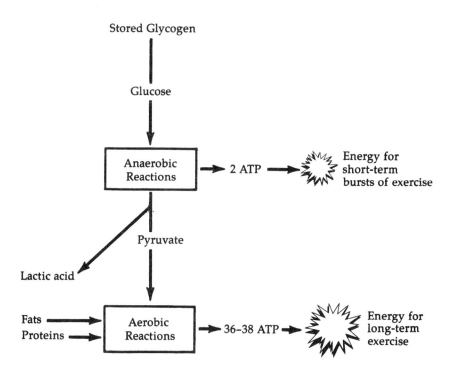

The Glucose Anaerobic Pathway

The first stage is called the anaerobic pathway, where glucose is broken down to a substance called *pyruvate*. When oxygen is not available, this pyruvate will be converted to lactic acid, forming 2 units of ATP. (When oxygen is available, pyruvate is broken down for energy in the aerobic pathway.)

There is a limit to the amount of lactic acid the body can tolerate. This is why anaerobic metabolism can only fuel exercise by itself for a short period of time (a few minutes). Lactic acid can be used for energy, but during anaerobic exercise it is produced faster than it can be used. When you break down glycogen rapidly, your body accumulates lactic acid and you feel fatigued faster.

The anaerobic pathway provides us with the energy for short, intense exercise such as sprinting. It also provides energy for the bursts which are common in sports like soccer, basketball, football and tennis.

The anaerobic pathway also contributes energy during prolonged exercise such as marathon running, when the level of intensity is suddenly increased (e.g., when climbing a hill, or sprinting). The bulk of the energy for such prolonged exercise must be aerobically supplied, but when the exercise intensity increases, there is a point where aerobic metabolism cannot meet the energy requirements of the exercise by itself. At this point, energy from the anaerobic pathway is pulled in to assist the aerobic pathway.

The Glucose Aerobic Pathway

As I said, the breakdown of glucose takes place in two stages, and the second stage is the aerobic pathway. You will recall that aerobic metabolism depends on a continuous supply of oxygen. When oxygen is made available to the muscles, pyruvate will be broken down far more efficiently for energy, without being converted to lactic acid. Pyruvate broken down with oxygen provides 36 to 38 ATP (18 to 19 times more immediate energy than if it had been broken down without oxygen). *How can you influence your body to break down glucose more efficiently?* One way is to control the intensity of the exercise so that sufficient oxygen will be continuously available to the muscles.

Capacities for exercise intensity and duration are inversely related: As distances increase, runners have to reduce their pace. (A marathon runner would have to run a slower average pace in his 26.2-mile race than if he were running a 10K. — a 10-kilometer race — which would be slower yet than if he were running a 5K., and so on.) Everyone has a maximum aerobic capacity, but can only perform at a certain percentage of that capacity for any given distance or time.

For example, a trained endurance runner can run a mile at 100% of his aerobic capacity. In a 5K., he can use about 95% of his aerobic capacity. In a 10K., he can average about 90% of his aerobic capacity. In the marathon, he can only use 60 to 80% of his aerobic capacity. His aerobic machinery simply cannot tolerate the same level of intensity as the distance increases.

Why not? Because he will outstrip his oxygen supply, rely more on anaerobically-supplied energy, and increasingly accumulate lactic acid. His legs will feel heavy and refuse to cooperate. He'll have to stop or slow down.

Even in shorter events, such as a 5K., pace becomes extremely important. If you go out too fast, too much lactic acid will accumulate and the advantage you gained with the early speed will be more than offset by your sub-par performance the rest of the race. This is what happened to the runner in the story at the beginning of the chapter.

In longer events, such as the marathon, I mentioned an

additional reason (besides lactic acid accumulation) why we cannot perform at close to our aerobic capacity for the whole race: During endurance exercise which exceeds an hour and a half, muscle glycogen stores become progressively depleted. When your muscle glycogen stores drop to low levels, you feel exhausted and must either stop exercising or continue at a much slower pace. We'll discuss glycogen depletion further in Chapters 4 and 5.

What about the other fuels?

Amino Acids

Amino acids from proteins are not a primary energy source during exercise. Their regular functions are for bodily growth and repair. However, when more efficient fuel sources are lacking, for instance because of fasting or a low carbohydrate diet, more protein will be used for energy during exercise.

Amino acids are an aerobic source of fuel, and require a continuous supply of oxygen. Therefore, amino acids can provide energy only during exercise of low to moderate intensity.

Fatty Acids

Fatty acids from fats are, like amino acids, an aerobic source of energy, and are not useful for high-intensity exercise. However, they are an extremely important energy source for endurance exercise, because, unlike carbohydrates, there is a virtually unlimited supply (and they are utilized more efficiently than amino acids).

The Aerobic/Anaerobic Combination

The aerobic and anaerobic pathways work together. At the beginning of exercise, it takes time for the heart and blood

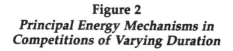

Figure 2
Principal Energy Mechanisms in Competitions of Varying Duration

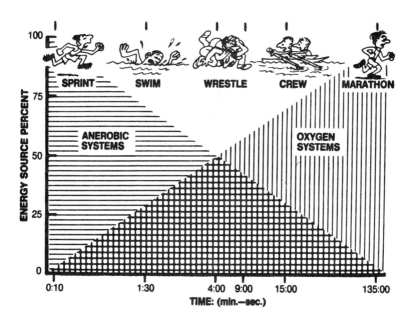

vessels to get oxygen-rich blood to the muscles and for the muscles to extract oxygen from the blood. (Thus the importance of a proper pre-event warm-up.) During this lag time (several minutes), the anaerobic pathway provides most of the energy for the exercise.

Eventually, the aerobic energy sources will in large part take over; but at any point in the exercise activity, when the intensity of the exercise becomes too great and the aerobic machinery alone can't keep up, the anaerobic pathway will be called on to meet the deficit.

In an event such as a half-mile run, the contributions of aerobic and anaerobic metabolism are about equal. As the distance increases, the contribution of aerobically produced energy increases. Ultimately, the energy dependence placed respectively on the aerobic and anaerobic pathways will determine whether you finish your event, how well you finish, and the intensity at which you perform throughout the event.

As we will see, what you eat and drink before and during the event will affect your ability to get the most out of your energy sources.

Chapter 2

The Golden Standard of Physical Fitness

Measuring Your Capacity to Use Oxygen

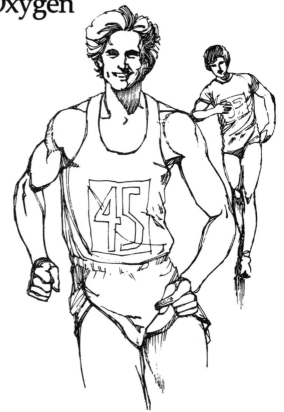

You and your buddy run and have almost identical times in the mile, and trade off leads in the 10K. You both decide to run a marathon, and train together for it by putting in many long, comfortable runs. After tapering off on your mileage, you both carbohydrate load for the event.

On the day of the marathon you run together for the first ten miles. Your buddy has a tough time keeping the pace after that but you feel good. Finally, he tells you to take off, and you leave your friend behind.

You finish the race with no problems and wait at the finish line. Finally, he walks in. "What happened?"

"When I hit the twenty-first mile I felt terrible," he said. "I could only walk."

Later, over dinner, you re-hash the race. "How come," he laments, "I can run with you in a 10K. but not in a marathon?"

We have seen the importance of oxygen for endurance exercise. We have also noted how lactic acid build-up can be a limiting factor on ability to perform. Because both of these factors are so important, we will now see how the capacity of an athlete to use oxygen, and the level at which his muscles accumulate lactic acid have both become standard measures, used to predict his capacity for performance.

Maximal Oxygen Consumption

The harder you exercise, the more oxygen you require. The amount of oxygen that your body uses is directly related to the intensity of the exercise.

However, there is a point beyond which your use of oxygen will not increase, even when the intensity of the exercise continues to increase. This value, at which your oxygen consumption plateaus, is called your maximal oxygen consumption (abbreviated $\dot{V}O_{2max}$). $\dot{V}O_{2max}$ is a scientific measurement of your aerobic capacity, and is regarded as the best criterion of endurance capacity and physical fitness. A person with a high $\dot{V}O_{2max}$ can exercise harder and longer than a person with a low $\dot{V}O_{2max}$.

A large person will use more total oxygen because he* has more oxygen-requiring tissue. To account for individual differences in size, $\dot{V}O_{2max}$ values factor in differences in body weight. A person's maximal oxygen usage (measured in liters per minute) is divided by his weight (measured in kilograms — one kilogram is equal to 2.2

---

*To avoid the awkwardness of either (1) avoiding singular personal pronouns, or (2) using "him/her," etc., the masculine form will be used unless the context calls for the feminine.

pounds). VO_{2max} values are expressed as: milliliters of oxygen used per kilogram of body weight per minute (abbreviated ml/kg/min).

Values for sedentary college age males and females are in the mid 40s and 30s ml/kg/min respectively. Endurance male athletes (runners, cyclists, triathletes, swimmers) generally have $\dot{V}O_{2max}$ values in the 60s, and elite male athletes have values in the 70s to 80s ml/kg/min. Female endurance athletes are usually in the 50s and elite female athletes are in the 60s to 70s ml/kg/min.

Your ultimate aerobic capacity seems to be genetically determined, but whether you reach your potential will depend on training. An untrained person can improve his $\dot{V}O_{2max}$ by up to 20% with endurance training.

We define endurance exercise as exercising for 3 to 5 days per week, for 20 to 60 minutes, at 50 to 80% of $\dot{V}O_{2max}$ (or 60 to 90% of maximum heart rate). Aerobic capacity peaks within 6 months to 2 years following the initiation of an endurance exercise program. However, even after your $\dot{V}O_{2max}$ has stopped increasing, you can continue to improve your performance. Why?

$\dot{V}O_{2max}$ and Performance

Very few athletes can exercise at their $\dot{V}O_{2max}$ for more than about 5 minutes. This means that most of the time we are exercising at a percentage of our aerobic capacity (e.g., 95% in a 5K., 60-80% in a marathon). Even when your VO_{2max} no longer increases, you can continue to improve by developing the ability to tax a higher percentage of your aerobic capacity.

In practical terms, this means that you can complete the same distance at a faster speed for the same effort. Whereas most marathon runners run at a pace which requires 60 to 80% of their $\dot{V}O_{2max}$, elite marathoners can run the distance at 90% of their VO_{2max}.

An example of one such athlete is Derek Clayton, who once held the world record in the marathon. His $\dot{V}O_{2max}$ was below that expected for a world record performer (69.7 ml/kg/min), but he was able to run at a pace which represented 88% of his aerobic capacity. (Training improvement does have its limits — the genetically endowed athlete who can work close to his $\dot{V}O_{2max}$ will continue to have the edge over the less endowed athlete.)

Women, non-athletes and athletes alike, have lower aerobic capacities than men. Women have less total hemoglobin and so the oxygen content of the blood delivered to their muscles is lower. They also have a lower muscle mass and can't use as much oxygen. In addition, a greater percentage of their body weight is fat.

When $\dot{V}O_{2max}$ is re-expressed relative to active muscle mass (rather than body weight), the differences between the sexes almost disappear. Though this implies that men and women may have the same endurance potential (a given muscle will get as much oxygen), women must still carry their entire body weight (less muscle carrying more fat), and their performance is affected accordingly.

The Anaerobic Threshold

The anaerobic threshold may explain why endurance training results in the ability to tax a higher percentage of your $\dot{V}O_{2max}$. It may also explain why some athletes can reach a higher percentage than others during endurance exercise.

The anaerobic threshold is the point where, as exercise intensity is increasing, glycogen is broken down more rapidly and lactic acid begins to accumulate (expressed as the percentage of $\dot{V}O_{2max}$).

Untrained people have anaerobic thresholds (begin to accumulate lactic acid) at about 50% of their $\dot{V}O_{2max}$. Trained people have anaerobic thresholds at about 70% of their $\dot{V}O_{2max}$. The increased exercise level for lactic acid accumulation means that the person can exercise at a higher percentage of $\dot{V}O_{2max}$. (Remember that increased glycogen breakdown causes the accumulation of lactic acid, with subsequent fatigue.)

To repeat, an athlete with an anaerobic threshold at 70% of his aerobic capacity should have a better endurance potential than an athlete with the same aerobic capacity but an anaerobic threshold at 60%. Again, the higher percentage indicates that he can work closer to his aerobic capacity without accumulating lactic acid.

Remember the two marathon runners in the story at the beginning of the chapter? Although they could run a 10K. together, the athlete with the higher anaerobic threshold performed better in the marathon. This is because he had a slower rate of muscle glycogen depletion, which enabled him to maintain a faster running speed throughout the entire race.

In contrast, a 10K. race does not last long enough to be limited by muscle glycogen depletion. We'll discuss this further in Chapter 3.

At this time it is still not clear whether genetics or training has the greatest influence over where lactic acid accumulates. And even though it's known that endurance training can increase the anaerobic threshold, we still do not know the exact training regimen that promotes the largest increases. One study* found significant increases when the exercise intensity for training was halfway between the participants' anaerobic threshold and their $\dot{V}O_{2max}$.

Your $\dot{V}O_{2max}$ and anaerobic threshold can be measured during a graded exercise test on a bicycle or treadmill. Anaerobic threshold must be measured — it can't be estimated from a graded exercise test or one and one-half mile run. Many sports medicine facilities, colleges and hospitals offer such tests.

* *J Appl Physiol*, 46:1039-1046, 1979

Chapter 3

What Determines Fuel Usage?

Your Body's Use of
Glycogen and Fat

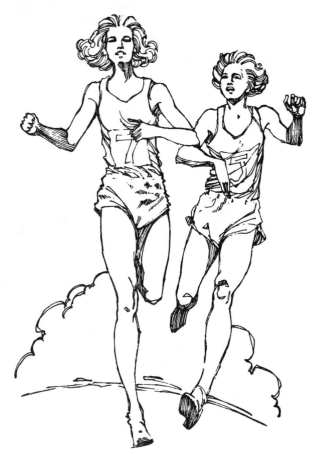

Two of my friends were competing in the same marathon. I expected them to finish in about the same time — based on their performances in other races and their comparable times during marathon training. One went out faster than she had planned and passed the half marathon mark five minutes ahead of schedule. The other woman came through the half marathon point right on her predicted pace. By 20 miles, the woman who had gone out slower passed the woman who had thought she was "putting money in the bank" by going out so fast.

The woman who paced herself finished comfortably and was several minutes ahead of her predicted time. The woman who went out too fast finished in agony, several minutes slower than her target time.

Your goal is to supply energy to the muscle and you have two major fuels — glycogen (your high octane fuel) and fat. A variety of factors determine which type of fuel your muscles will use during exercise. These include: the intensity of the exercise, the duration of the exercise, your fitness level, and the composition of your diet.

Intensity

The intensity of the exercise is particularly important in determining your muscles' energy source. Exercise that is intense in nature and lasts a fairly short time (such as sprinting) depends principally on the anaerobic pathway for energy. For such exercise, only glucose, derived principally from the breakdown of muscle glycogen, can be used for fuel.

As you will recall from Chapter 1, glucose used aerobically (during exercise of low to moderate intensity) will provide 16 to 19 times the energy of glucose used anaerobically. Thus the use of the anaerobic energy source results in muscle glycogen being used 18 to 19 times faster than where the glucose is used aerobically. This rapid rate of glycogen breakdown will also occur where high intensity exercise (i.e., over 70% $\dot{V}O_{2max}$) is interspersed with continuous exercise utilizing both aerobic and anaerobic metabolism to meet energy needs. (An example would be a sprint during a marathon.)

Exercise of low to moderate intensity (up to 60% of $\dot{V}O_{2max}$) can be fueled aerobically, primarily by fatty acids. Once you start exercising, specific hormones secreted during exercise cause your fat (adipose) tissue to release fatty acids into the bloodstream. These, combined with fat pools within the muscle, supply most of the energy demands for exercise of low to moderate intensity. Glycogen and blood glucose supply the rest.

Fat can be used generally as fuel until lactic acid begins to accumulate. Beyond this point glycogen is used more heavily, because lactic acid hinders the mobilization of fatty acids from the adipose tissue. This shift in muscle fuel from fat to glycogen is partly due to the accumulation of lactic acid during high intensity exercise. When lactic acid accumulates, the muscles must rely more on muscle glycogen for energy.

Generally, exercise above 70% of an endurance athlete's aerobic capacity (remember that most trained people have anaerobic thresholds at about 70% of their $\dot{V}O_{2max}$) will cause faster glycogen depletion than if the athlete exercises at a lower intensity. Muscle glycogen depletion is a well recognized limitation to endurance performance (and will be discussed further in Chapters 4 and 5).

At lower intensities (below 70% of $\dot{V}O_{2max}$), where exercise can be fueled by fatty acid, glycogen is spared, and you can exercise for a longer period of time. But when intensity increases, fat metabolism cannot provide enough energy (calories) to support the more intense level of exercise.

A word on pacing. Because intense exercise requires glycogen as fuel, whereas moderate exercise can be fueled by essentially limitless fatty acids, any sparing of muscle glycogen will result in increased endurance. This is the physiological basis for choosing a pace that can be maintained for long periods of time.

You use more glycogen than necessary by going out too fast in a race and/or by continuing at a pace that is too fast. To put it another way, your maximum long-term effective pace will be at the speed (intensity) which relies mainly on fatty acid metabolism and avoids lactic acid build-up and glycogen depletion.

Duration

The duration of exercise also determines whether the fuel used will be predominantly glycogen or fat. As the time spent exercising increases, the contribution of fat to the energy demands increases. Fat may supply as much as 60 to 70% of the energy needed during moderate intensity exercise lasting from 4 to 6 hours. As the duration of the exercise increases, and glycogen stores are depleted, the intensity of the exercise must decrease, as you need to depend more on fat metabolism.

Keep in mind that it takes from 30 to 60 minutes of continuous exercise for fat to be available as fuel in the form of free fatty acids. This means that muscle glycogen is the predominant fuel for most forms of exercise.

This does not mean that a person needs to work out for an hour to lose body fat. When the workout creates a caloric deficit, the body will pull from its fat stores at a later time to make up that caloric deficit. So, if 200 calories burned off in a 30-minute workout represent a caloric deficit for that day, those 200 calories will eventually come from body fat.

Fitness Level

Your fitness level will directly influence what type of fuel your muscles use during exercise — training increases your ability to perform aerobically at more intense levels of exercise. This means that with training you can use fat as a primary energy source at higher levels, when your body otherwise would be calling more on your glycogen stores.

Untrained people break down glycogen faster and so accumulate more lactic acid in their blood at a given workload than trained people, and so will use more glycogen and less fat as fuel. Endurance training results in a greater release of fatty acids from the adipose tissue

Figure 3
Relationship Between Distance and Energy Sources

Distance of Race	O$_2$ Consumption (% of MaxVO$_2$)	Glycogen Contribution	Fat
Marathon	75%	70%	30%
30 Kilo	78%	70%	30%
20 Kilo	80%	70%	30%
15 Kilo	81%	75%	25%
10 Kilo	83%	80%	20%
5 Kilo	90%	95%	5%
800 meters	100%	100%	0%

and increases the capacity of the aerobic machinery in your muscles to use fat.

Also, endurance training increases the capacity of your muscles to store glycogen. Thus training confers a double performance advantage — your muscle glycogen stores are higher prior to exercise and you deplete them at a slower rate.

Let's compare an unfit person to a fit person. The cardiovascular system of an unfit person cannot supply as much oxygen to his muscles, and his muscles cannot extract as much oxygen. (The ability of your heart to deliver oxygen, and of your muscles to extract the oxygen, together determine your aerobic capacity.) This means that the anaerobic pathway will be pulled in to assist and lactic acid will accumulate at a lower level of work. (As mentioned before, lactic acid suppresses the mobilization of fat from the adipose tissue.)

The muscles then shift the balance of their glycogen/fat utilization to use relatively more glycogen as a fuel. The result: In an unfit person, glycogen depletion occurs at a faster rate.

This is another way of saying what I emphasized earlier: The choice of fuel during exercise depends on your aerobic capacity (ability of your heart to supply oxygen) and your anaerobic threshold (level at which lactic acid build-up starts to inhibit your muscles' ability to use fatty acids aerobically).

Let's compare two athletes — one has a $\dot{V}O_{2max}$ of 70 ml/kg/min, the other a $\dot{V}O_{2max}$ of 60 ml/kg/min. They both have anaerobic thresholds at 70% of their respective $\dot{V}O_{2max}$'s. The athlete with the higher aerobic capacity can use fat for higher intensity exercise than the athlete with the lower aerobic capacity. The athlete with the lower $\dot{V}O_{2max}$ will deplete his glycogen stores faster.

On the other hand, if the athlete with the lower $\dot{V}O_{2max}$ trained himself to the point where his anaerobic threshold came at a higher percentage of his $\dot{V}O_{2max}$, he could make up the genetic difference. If their anaerobic thresholds occurred at the same absolute workload (e.g., when they both ran 10 miles per hour), they would tend to have the same endurance potential.

Diet

The relative amounts of carbohydrate and fat in your diet will affect the amounts of glycogen and fat you use during exercise. If your diet is high in carbohydrate, you'll have more glycogen to use as fuel. If your diet is high in fat, you'll have to use more fat as fuel. Though fat can be a primary energy source, this does not mean that you should "fat load" — even the leanest athletes have more fat stored than they'll ever need.

Your goal is to increase your fat utilization — not your body fat. You can do this far more effectively and healthfully by endurance training than by eating a high-fat diet. We'll discuss this further in Chapter 6.

If you eat a high-carbohydrate diet during training your muscles will store more glycogen. Maximum glycogen storage depends on a combination of diet and training (endurance training permits greater glycogen storage). Carbohydrate should provide 60 to 70% of your calories during training to ensure optimal muscle glycogen stores. We'll discuss this further in the next chapter.

Chapter 4

Recommended Training Diet
Eating for Both Health and Performance

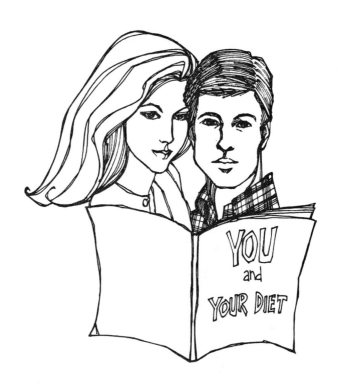

A friend of mine was training for a 200-mile bicycle ride. A week before the event, he headed out for a hilly 100-mile workout. He noticed that his legs felt stiff and heavy but thought he'd loosen up on the ride. He struggled to complete the first climb, standing up in his lowest gear on a grade he could normally surmount with ease. At the top of the hill, he gave up and headed home.

When we met over dinner that evening, he was about to give up on his 200-mile attempt. I told him to rest a day and eat a high-carbohydrate diet while tapering his training for the remainder of the week. He finished the 200-mile ride in his best time ever.

My friend had succumbed to training glycogen depletion.

To build up glycogen stores, or even to maintain existing glycogen stores during intensive training requires a carbohydrate-rich diet. To maintain general health, however, any diet should be balanced — a "prudent diet," as defined by the national guidelines. The Food Exchange System plan provides a simple guide for meeting basic nutritional requirements, which can be readily adapted to meet the special requirements of athletic training and competition.

Glycogen Stores and Training

Most people think that muscle glycogen depletion only occurs during prolonged endurance exercise like marathon running. However, glycogen depletion may also be a gradual process, occurring over repeated days of heavy training, where muscle glycogen is used faster than it is replaced. When this happens, your glycogen stores drop lower with each successive day, and your workouts become more difficult and less enjoyable.

A tell-tale sign of training glycogen depletion is when your normal exercise intensity is difficult to maintain. Your performance gradually deteriorates, and even an easy workout causes fatigue. A sudden weight loss of several pounds (due to glycogen and water loss) often accompanies training glycogen depletion.

Training glycogen depletion occurs so often that most athletes don't even think it's unusual. It's normal to be tired after several days of high intensity workouts, especially if you're exercising several hours a day. However, if you're always tired, your diet may be at fault.

When you don't consume enough carbohydrate, and/or don't take days off to rest, you're a prime candidate.

Dietary Carbohydrate and Glycogen

Training glycogen depletion can be prevented by a carbohydrate-rich diet, and periodic rest days to give the muscles time to rebuild their stores. By eating a carbohydrate-rich diet, you can maintain adequate muscle glycogen stores and exercise harder and longer with less fatigue.

Carbohydrate is essential for glycogen synthesis, and it should provide at least 60% of your total calories. The typical American diet (46% carbohydrate) doesn't supply enough carbohydrate to replace the glycogen you lose during heavy training. On such a diet a training athlete is susceptible to fatigue, when muscle glycogen stores are depleted. On the other hand, a high-carbohydrate diet (70% of calories) can restore muscle glycogen to normal levels in 24 hours, restoring endurance even during repeated days of high intensity exercise.

One study* compared glycogen synthesis on a 40% carbohydrate diet (300 to 350 grams of carbohydrate) to a 70% carbohydrate diet (500 to 600 grams of carbohydrate). On the low-carbohydrate diet, muscle glycogen levels dropped lower with each successive day of training, until the athletes couldn't perform even moderate intensity exercise. The high-carbohydrate diet almost completely replaced the muscle glycogen stores from day to day, allowing the athletes to continue heavy training.

A diet containing 8 grams of carbohydrate per kilogram per day (about 70% carbohydrate) is recommended when you're exercising hard (70% of VO_{2max} or more) for several hours or more daily. However, if you're exercising for an hour or less, a diet containing 6 grams of carbohydrate per kilogram per day (about 60% carbohydrate) is sufficient to replenish your glycogen stores. By keeping your carbohydrate intake high, you can guard against the gradual depletion of muscle glycogen that can cause fatigue after repeated days of hard workouts.

A Prudent Diet — Emphasis on Carbohydrates

In addition to providing adequate muscle glycogen stores, a prudent diet should help to prevent heart disease, stroke and cancer. You can meet these objectives by following the U.S. Dietary Goals established by the U.S. Senate Select Committee on Nutrition and Human Needs. In this diet, complex carbohydrates provide approximately 48% of calories, sugar not more than 8 to 12% of calories, protein 12% of calories, and fat no more than 30% of calories. (See sample meal plans in the Appendix.)

In addition to generally promoting optimum health, this high-carbohydrate, low-fat diet, will optimize muscle glycogen stores, unless you are in heavy training. If you are, and you want to increase your carbohydrate intake to 70%, you should reduce your fat intake to 20% or less. (See Chapter 5.) When you eat a 70% carbohydrate diet, you may increase your sugar consumption, but at least 48% of your calories should continue to come from complex carbohydrates.

(There are two basic types of carbohydrates: complex carbohydrates — fruits, vegetables, whole grain breads and cereals, pasta, grains and beans; and refined carbohydrates — sugars and sweets.)

Complex CHO vs Sugar

Sugar and complex carbohydrates (starch) are grouped together as carbohydrates because they have a chemical similarity. All carbohydrates are made up of one or more simple sugars — the three most common being glucose, fructose and galactose. The simple sugar glucose connected to fructose forms sucrose, or table sugar. When more than two glucose molecules are connected, they become a complex carbohydrate. Complex carbohydrates contain anywhere from 300 to 1,000 or more glucose units linked together. Our body uses both the sugars and starches for energy.

There appears to be no difference in glycogen storage between complex carbohydrates and refined carbohydrates. However, complex carbohydrates should be emphasized since they provide vitamins, minerals, and fiber with their calories.

Food Exchange System

In practical terms, a high-carbohydrate diet can be obtained by using a Food Exchange System. The Exchange lists recommended here are the basis of a meal planning system developed by a committee of the American Dietetic Association and the American Diabetes Association.

There are six exchange lists: meat, vegetables, fruit, starch/bread, milk and fat. Each lists foods that have about the same amount of carbohydrate, protein, fat, and calories. Any food on a list can be exchanged or traded for any other food on the same list.

Figure 4
Food Group Exchanges

Starch/Bread/Grains (80 calories)

15 grams carbohydrate
3 grams protein
0 grams fat

½ cup pasta, barley, cooked
  cereal
⅓ cup rice or dried cooked
  peas/beans
½ cup corn, peas, winter squash
1 small (3 oz.) baked potato
4-6 crackers
1 slice bread or 6" tortilla
½ bagel, english muffin, pita
¾ cup dry flaked cereal
3 cups popcorn, no oil or butter
¾ oz. pretzels

Meat and Meat Alternatives
(55-100 calories)

0 grams carbohydrate
7 grams protein
3-8 grams fat

1 oz. poultry, fish, beef, pork,
  lamb, etc.
¼ cup tuna, salmon, cottage
  cheese
2 tbsp. peanut butter
1 egg
1 oz. cheese
tofu (2½" x 2¾" x 1")

Vegetables (25 calories)

5 grams carbohydrate
2 grams protein
0 grams fat

½ cup cooked vegetables
1 cup raw vegetables
½ cup tomato or vegetable juice

Milk (90-150 calories)

12 grams carbohydrate
8 grams protein
0-5 grams fat

1 cup milk: non-fat, low-fat, 1%,
  whole
1 cup yogurt: non-fat, low-fat,
  1%, whole

Fruit (60 calories)

15 grams carbohydrate
0 grams protein
0 grams fat

1 medium fresh fruit
1 cup berries or melon
½ cup canned fruit (without
  sugar)
½ cup fruit juice
¼ cup dried fruit

Fat (45 calories)

0 grams carbohydrate
0 grams protein
5 grams fat

1 tsp. margarine, oil, butter,
  mayonnaise
2 tsp. diet margarine, diet
  mayonnaise
1 tbs. salad dressing, cream
  cheese, cream, nuts
2 tbs. diet salad dressing, sour
  cream
1 slice bacon

Figure 5
Training Diet Meal Plans

Food Group	Number of Exchanges					
	Calorie Level					
	1,500	2,000	2,500	3,000	3,500	4,000
Milk	3	3	4	4	4	4
Meat	5	5	5	5	6	6
Fruit	5	6	7	9	10	12
Vegetable	3	3	3	5	6	7
Grain	7	11	16	18	20	24
Fat	2	3	5	6	8	10

Figure 5 contains plans for different calorie levels from 1,500 to 4,000. These exchange plans are designed to supply about 60% carbohydrate, 15 to 20% protein, and less than 25% fat. Since the milk, bread, and fruit exchanges have the most carbohydrate per serving, they are emphasized. These exchange plans will meet the carbohydrate needs for most workout schedules.

Sugary foods, such as cakes, cookies, pies, soft drinks, and candy can supply additional carbohydrate but are low in most other nutrients.

There's no harm in eating high-carbohydrate "empty calories" to supply needed calories after you have made sure you've met your nutrient needs. But don't just eat a small number of servings of complex carbohydrates and then fill up on sweets to meet your carbohydrate needs. You will be wise to give yourself a safety margin with extra servings of nutritious complex carbohydrates.

Commercial Carbohydrate Supplements

Some people train so heavily that they have difficulty eating enough food to obtain the amount of carbohydrate needed for optimal performance. This can happen for several reasons.

Often the stress of hard training can reduce the appetite, taking the pleasure out of eating and tending to reduce the amount eaten. Also, consuming a large volume of food can cause gastrointestinal distress and interfere with training. Finally, some people spend so much time training that there aren't many rest hours available for replenishment.

Those who have difficulty consuming enough carbohydrate can use a commercial high-carbohydrate supplement. These products do not replace regular food but are designed to supply supplemental calories and carbohydrate. If you have no difficulty eating enough carbohydrate-rich food, however, these products are unnecessary.

These products should be consumed before or after exercise. Their carbohydrate content is too high for use as fluid replacement drinks during exercise.

Nutrition Counseling

If you want individualized nutrition counseling, consult a registered dietitian (credentials abbreviated: R.D.). A registered dietitian is a legally recognized health care professional who is educated in nutrition and food science. R.D.'s must follow specific coursework and obtain a

Figure 6
High-Carbohydrate Beverage Comparison Chart

Beverage	Flavors	Carbohydrate Type	Percent Carbohydrate	Serving Size (ounce)	Carbohydrate gram/ounce	Sodium mg/ounce
GatorLode™ The Quaker Oats Company	Lemon, Citrus, Banana	Maltodextrin and Glucose	20	12	5.9	7.9
Exceed® Ross Laboratories	Golden, Punch, Fruit Punch	Maltodextrin and Sucrose	24	32	7.1	14.7
Carboplex® Unipro, Inc.	Plain	Maltodextrin	23	8	6.8	0
Carbo Energizer™ Weider Health & Fitness, Inc.	Orange	Maltodextrin	25	8	7.4	16.3
Carbo Power™ Nature's Best Food Supplements	Lemon/Lime	Maltodextrin and High Fructose Corn Syrup	18	16	5.3	6.3
Carbo Cooler® Sport Beverage Company	Grape, Orange, Fruit Punch	Maltodextrin and Fructose	21	16	6.2	0
Paragon Fast Recovery™ Avadyne, Inc.	Plain	Maltodextrin and Fructose	25	8	7.4	0

Source: Used by permission of the Gatorade Company.

bachelor's degree from an accredited university. They have an internship, take a national certification exam, and maintain their registration through continued professional education.

Beware of self-proclaimed nutrition "experts" who promote questionable foods, supplements, and fad diets. The title "nutritionist" can be used by anyone regardless of training. Only the R.D. has the educational background and clinical training to be an effective counselor. You can find an R.D. by requesting a referral from your physician, contacting the nutrition department of a hospital, clinic or community health agency, or by checking in the phone book under dietitians, nutritionists, and weight control (remember to look for the R.D. behind the name).

There are registered dietitians who specialize in sports nutrition. They usually belong to the Sports and Cardiovascular Nutrition Group (abbreviated SCAN) of the American Dietetic Association.

Chapter 5

Carbohydrate Loading

Filling Your Tank with High Octane Fuel

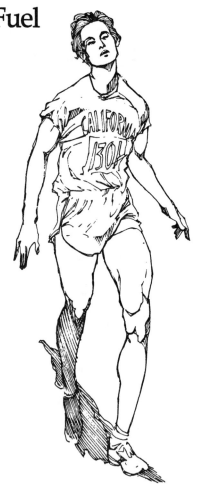

I thought muscle glycogen depletion was a crackpot theory until I experienced it.

It was my third marathon. I had averaged eight-minute miles all the way out and passed the 15 and 18 mile markers with no problems — feeling fine.

At the twentieth mile I felt weak and had problems lifting my legs. It took a concerted effort to run. By the 21st mile, 2:40 out, that was it. I couldn't run. There was nothing left. I felt excruciating pain in my thighs. Everything hurt. Walking hurt, but it was possible. I walked the last five miles. Each time I tried to run, I couldn't lift my legs. Even to try was extremely painful.

Later, after the fact, I thought that it had just been a lack of will power.

In my next marathon, though, I encountered the same situation. After about three hours, I just couldn't run slow enough. Couldn't even shuffle. I walked in again.

After that I became a firm believer in "the wall."

As originally developed, the glycogen-loading regimen was difficult to follow, and athletes tended either to give up on it, or to compromise their training schedule. As now revised, it involves no hardship, and is just as effective. But the basic ground rules must be understood.

The Wall

During endurance exercise which exceeds 90 minutes, such as running, your muscle glycogen stores become progressively lower. When they drop to critically low levels (the point of "glycogen depletion"), you are exhausted and must either stop exercising or drastically reduce your pace. Marathon runners frequently refer to muscle glycogen depletion as "hitting the wall" — that point in the marathon, usually around the 20-mile mark, where it is common, and running becomes virtually impossible.

Glycogen Stores

One obvious way to improve your endurance then, if you're exercising longer than for an hour and a half, is to increase your muscle glycogen stores. The higher your pre-exercise muscle glycogen level, the greater your endurance potential. This is the rationale behind carbohydrate loading. When done properly, carbohydrate loading can double your muscle glycogen stores.

Let's take a practical look at what this means. If you eat a normal American diet (46% carbohydrate), you can exercise hard (at 75% of your aerobic capacity) for one and one-half to two hours before muscle glycogen depletion. After following the carbohydrate loading regimen (70% carbohydrate with tapered training), you can exercise at the same intensity for three hours and possibly longer. This means that carbohydrate loading can buy you an additional hour or more of high intensity exercise.

However, carbohydrate loading is only effective when you follow a specific week-long diet and exercise plan.

Carbohydrate Loading

The Original Diet

As originally practiced*, carbohydrate loading was hard to follow because of the extreme diet shifts during the last week of training. Beginning with the seventh day before competition, you would exercise hard for 90 minutes, specifically working the muscles you used in your event. You would continue doing this for the next three days, and you would eat a low-carbohydrate diet (below 40% carbohydrate), the purpose being to further lower your muscle glycogen levels. Then for the three days immediately prior to competition, you would switch to a carbohydrate-rich diet (at least 70% carbohydrate) — and finally rest. The depleted muscles would in effect soak up the glycogen to the point of maximum storage. For many years, this week-long sequence was considered the best way to insure maximum glycogen storage.

However, the low-carbohydrate diet component of that old technique caused many people to quit the regimen, or avoid it altogether. Three days on a low-carbohydrate diet can cause low blood sugar (hypoglycemia) and increased blood acids from fat breakdown (ketosis), with associated

*Acta Physiol Scand, 71:140-150, 1967

nausea, fatigue, dizziness and irritability. Attempting to train on such a low-carbohydrate diet is a sheer test of will power, when muscle glycogen stores are at abnormally low levels. Also, the sudden switching from a low to a high-carbohydrate diet proved to be too cumbersome for many athletes, and they couldn't stick with the week-long sequence.

The Revised Diet

A revised version* of carbohydrate loading has been developed which eliminates many of the problems associated with the classical routine. Beginning with the sixth day before competition, you exercise hard (70 to 75% $\dot{V}O_{2max}$) for 90 minutes. On that day and the next two days, you eat a normal American diet — 5 grams of carbohydrate per kilogram of body weight per day (about 50% carbohydrate). For the second and third days, decrease your training to 40 minutes (still at 70-75% $\dot{V}O_{2max}$). On the next two days, you eat a high carbohydrate diet, 10 grams of carbohydrate per kilogram per day (still about 70% carbohydrate), and reduce your training to 20 minutes. Finally, you rest the day before competition, while maintaining the high-carbohydrate diet.

This modified sequence results in muscle glycogen levels equal to those provided by the classical regimen. However, the new routine eliminates the misery created by the low-carbohydrate diet and requires only one major dietary change — switching from an average American diet to a high-carbohydrate diet (the same diet you eat during heavy training).

Why Do Your Muscles Store Glycogen?

The classical carbohydrate loading technique used a low-carbohydrate diet because it was believed that this

*Int Sports Med, 2:114-118, 1981

Figure 7
Training and Diet Regimen for Glycogen Loading

	Day 1	Day 2	Day 3	Day 4	Day 5	Day 6	Day 7
TRAINING	90 Min. 70-75% $\dot{V}O_{2max}$	40 Min. 70-75% $\dot{V}O_{2max}$	40 Min. 70-75% $\dot{V}O_{2max}$	20 Min. 70-75% $\dot{V}O_{2max}$	20 Min. 70-75% $\dot{V}O_{2max}$	Rest	EVENT
EATING	50% Carbohy- drate 5 gm/kg	50% Carbohy- drate 5 gm/kg	50% Carbohy- drate 5 gm/kg	70% Carbohy- drate 10 gm/kg	70% Carbohy- drate 10 gm/kg	70% Carbohy- drate 10 gm/kg	EVENT

was necessary to achieve the maximum levels of muscle glycogen — that you had to absolutely deplete your glycogen stores right before you built them up. Now we know that exercise is the primary stimulus for increased muscle glycogen synthesis, and accomplishes the necessary lowering, leading to the glycogen build-up when the muscles have the chance. Tapering your training and eating a high-carbohydrate diet gives them this opportunity.

Since exercise is the primary stimulus for high muscle glycogen stores, you need to be endurance trained or carbohydrate loading won't work. If you're unfit and try to carbohydrate load, your muscles won't store more than their usual amount of glycogen. Even without carbohydrate loading, rested elite marathoners have muscle glycogen levels twice as high as normal, equal to the levels found in the carbohydrate loaded muscle of an average athlete. Elite endurance athletes probably won't benefit from the carbohydrate loading technique.

Selecting Food

When you eat an average American diet, you consume about 350 grams of carbohydrate per day (based on a total daily intake of 2,800 or more kcals), and get 50% of your calories from carbohydrate. To get a high-carbohydrate diet (about 70% of calories) from the same daily calorie total, you need to consume about 500 to 600 grams (2,000 to 2,400 calories) of carbohydrate. Exceeding 600 grams won't result in proportionately greater muscle glycogen stores.

To obtain a high-carbohydrate diet, you will need to eat more carbohydrate-rich foods than you eat during training. Cereals, breads, pasta, beans, rice, potatoes, corn, pancakes, and other starchy foods are the primary sources of carbohydrate. Other good sources include fruits, vegetables, milk, yogurt, ice milk and milkshakes and high sugar foods such as cakes, cookies, pies, soft drinks and candy.

If you have difficulty obtaining enough carbohydrate, you can consider taking a high-carbohydrate commercial supplement (see Figure 6 on page 37). For example, 24 ounces of GatorLode® provides 140 grams of carbohydrate and 24 ounces of Exceed High Carbohydrate Source® provides 170 grams of carbohydrate.

Maintain Nutritional Balance

Don't ignore your nutritional needs during carbohydrate loading. As followed by some athletes, the diet is deficient in certain vitamins and minerals necessary for peak performance and good health.

When you emphasize any dietary component, and particularly when refined carbohydrates are emphasized, your diet can easily be deficient. A high sugar intake can also result in gastrointestinal distress in the form of cramps,

Figure 8
Sample Glycogen Loading Menu 1

Breakfast
1 cup orange juice
1 cup oatmeal, with
1 banana
1 cup low-fat milk
2 slices wheat bread, with
1 tsp. margarine

Lunch	**Snack**
2 slices rye bread	8 graham crackers
3 oz. turkey	1 cup low-fat milk
1 oz. mozzarella cheese, with	1 apple
lettuce, tomato, mustard	
1 tsp. mayonnaise	
1 cup apple juice	
1 orange	
1 cup lemon sherbet	

Dinner	**Snack**
2 cups spaghetti	6 cups popcorn,
⅔ cup tomato sauce, with	air popped
mushrooms	
2 tbl. Parmesan cheese	
4 slices French bread	
2 tsp. margarine	
½ cup broccoli	
½ cup ice cream, with	
¾ cup strawberies	

Sample menu contains approximately 3,000 calories: 518 grams of carbohydrate.

Figure 9
Sample Glycogen Loading Menu 2

Breakfast

2 cups corn flakes
1 cup non-fat milk
2 cups orange juice (frozen)
3 slices cracked wheat bread
3 tsp. jelly

Snack

2 large bananas

Lunch

6 slices cracked wheat bread
3 oz turkey
3 oz. low-fat American cheese
2 cups apple juice

Snack

2 almond granola bars

Dinner

3 cups spaghetti with
non-meat sauce
2 medium rolls
2 tbl. margarine
1 cup green beans
1 cup non-fat milk
2 large oranges

Snack

2 large apples

Sample menu contains approximately 4,000 calories: 607 grams of carbohydrate.

nausea, diarrhea and bloating. You should stress complex carbohydrates over sweets for carbohydrate loading (as well as good health in general), because they provide nutrients with their calories.

Carbohydrate loading is not synonymous with overeating. Though the contribution of carbohydrate in your diet increases, your total caloric intake should remain the same.

Exercise

There are several things to keep in mind when you use carbohydrate loading. First, the exercise to deplete your glycogen stores must be the same as your own competitive event, because glycogen stores are specific to the muscle groups used. For example, a cyclist needs to deplete his stores by cycling rather than by running.

Second, it is essential that you decrease your training, or rest the three days prior to competition. Too much exercise will use too much of your stored glycogen and defeat the purpose of the entire process. This final three days, when you rest or barely exercise, is the real "loading" phase of the regimen.

Limitations

There are several side effects of carbohydrate loading that may make it inappropriate for some people. For each gram of glycogen stored, additional water is stored. Some people note a feeling of stiffness and heaviness associated with the increased glycogen storage. Once you start exercising, however, these sensations will work out.

If you have or are at risk for developing heart disease, diabetes and/or high blood triglycerides, you may have problems if you carbohydrate load. When in doubt, check with your doctor before attempting this regimen.

Remember that carbohydrate loading will only help for continuous exercise lasting more than an hour and a half. Greater than usual muscle glycogen stores won't enable you to exercise harder during exercise which lasts less than 90 minutes. Also, the stiffness and heaviness due to increased glycogen stores can hurt your performance during shorter competitions.

Also, keep in mind that carbohydrate loading enables you to maintain high intensity exercise longer, but will not affect your pace for the first hour of exercise. You won't be able to go out faster, but you'll be able to maintain your pace longer*.

*J *Appl Physiol*, 31:203-206, 1971

Chapter 6

Fat
Friend or Foe?

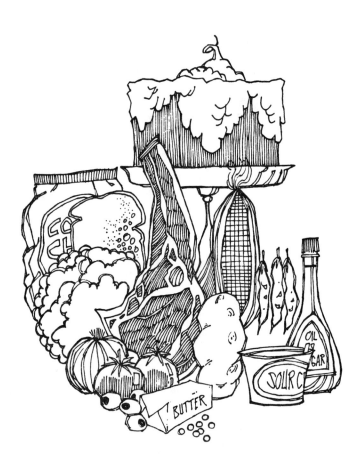

Wednesday night I visited a friend who planned to run a marathon on Saturday. He was cooking dinner, consisting of steak, a baked potato with sour cream, vegetable smothered in butter, a salad with lots of dressing and bread. For dessert he planned cake. While he was cooking he ate a half a bag of corn chips.

"What are you getting ready for?" I asked him.

He replied, "I'm carbohydrate loading."

"No you're not," I said. "You're fat loading."

Fat is definitely out of fashion. We fight fat to look good, and we are increasingly aware of the health risks of high-fat diets. But fat plays a positive role in endurance exercise. In fact, a prime purpose of training is to increase our ability to use fat for energy.

The Importance of Fat

The importance of being able to use fat for fuel can be illustrated by comparing elite with average marathon runners. Most average marathon runners dread the experience of "hitting the wall." When elite runners have been questioned, however, most say that they don't have to worry about it. Why the difference?

As I said in the previous chapter, "hitting the wall" means muscle glycogen depletion. It occurs within 90-120 minutes of exercise at 75% $\dot{V}O_{2max}$. The elite marathoner escapes "the wall" because he runs the race so fast, before his glycogen stores are depleted. His exceptionally high $\dot{V}O_{2max}$ and anaerobic threshold both enable him to run marathons in close to two hours. He also uses more fat and thus spares glycogen in the process.

The elite marathoner also does not "hit the wall" because he is able to conserve his muscle glycogen stores. There is a limit to the maximum amount of glycogen that anyone can store, less than the energy required to run a marathon, so the difference cannot be attributed to a difference in stores. It relates to the differences in the rate at which athletes deplete glycogen. Elite athletes use fat and spare glycogen better than average athletes, due to their higher $\dot{V}O_{2max}$'s and anaerobic thresholds.

Fat is the most concentrated source of food energy, supplying more than twice as many calories by weight as protein or carbohydrate. Fats are our only source of linoleic acid, an essential nutrient required for growth and skin maintenance. Fats are also the source of fat-soluble vitamins. Fats make our food taste better. Fats also keep us from getting hungry for a longer period of time between meals.

Whereas our total glycogen stores (in muscle and liver) amount to only about 2,000 calories, every pound of fat supplies 3,500 calories. Fat is the major, if not always most important, fuel for light to moderate intensity exercise. However, even though fat makes significant energy contributions during longer-term aerobic exercise, no attempt should be made to store fat (as you can store glycogen), because more fat is stored than is ever needed.

Fat in the Diet

The average American diet supplies 37% of the calories from fat. All evidence suggests that this is too much — either for endurance athletes or sedentary people. It increases your risk of developing heart disease (our nation's number one killer), stroke and cancer. A high-fat diet also contributes to obesity, which is associated with a wide range of health problems.

Fat is present, but not separately visible in dairy products (particularly cheese, ice-cream and whole milk), meat, eggs, nuts, and fried foods. Other dietary sources are more clearly visible (e.g., margarine, butter, mayonnaise, salad dressing, oil and sour cream). You can decrease your fat intake by selecting low-fat dairy products (e.g., low-fat milk, and yogurt) and low-fat protein foods (e.g., chicken, fish, and beans), and by limiting your use of visible fat.

Fats are categorized as either saturated or unsaturated (including polyunsaturated and monounsaturated), with differing chemical make-up, and differing effects on bodily function and health. Saturated fat is solid at room temperature and is derived mainly from animal sources. Unsaturated fat is liquid at room temperature and is found mainly in plant sources. (Palm and coconut oils are exceptions — they are highly saturated vegetable fats.)

Saturated fats should comprise no more than 10% of your caloric intake, because saturated fat has been associated with increased cholesterol levels in the blood. A high blood cholesterol level is one of the three major controllable risk factors for heart disease (along with smoking and high blood pressure). Foods with high percentages of monounsaturated and polyunsaturated fats (e.g., canola, olive, corn and soy oil, and derivative margarines) should be substituted for those with high percentages of saturated fats (e.g., butter).

When choosing meat, your total fat, saturated fat and cholesterol consumption can be reduced by selecting lean meats, poultry and fish, and trimming off any visible fat. Cut down on butter, lard, shortening, salad dressing, oils and fried foods. When substituting margarine and oil for butter, keep in mind that they are still high in fat and calories. When using oil, use vegetable oils such as corn, safflower, canola and sunflower. Substitute non-fat and low-fat milk for whole milk, and low-fat dairy products for high-fat dairy products. Be more aware of the hidden fat in foods such as hamburger, cheese, ice cream, granola, french fries, bakery goods, eggs, avocados, chips, nuts, and many highly processed foods.

Using Fat to Conserve Glycogen

Also, if you eat more fat, you'll eat less carbohydrate. (Remember that you always want to optimize your muscle glycogen stores when preparing for endurance exercise.) Muscle glycogen stores cannot be adequately maintained on a high-fat diet.

Glycogen provides more calories (energy) per liter of oxygen than does fat. (If we calculate the efficiency of utilization for glucose, we learn that glucose delivers 5.01 calories per liter of oxygen and fat delivers 4.65 calories per liter of oxygen.) So, when less oxygen becomes available (as one approaches one's $\dot{V}O_{2max}$), it is a distinct advantage for the muscles to be able to use glycogen because less oxygen is required.

Increasing Ability to Use Fat

I pointed out that there is no training advantage to increasing your body fat stores. But there is an important advantage to increasing your body's ability to burn fat as fuel. The ability to use fat will spare muscle glycogen; and also, after your limited stores of glycogen, fat is your most efficient fuel.

Endurance training causes two major adaptations that increase fat utilization. First, endurance training results in a greater release of free fatty acids from the fat tissue. Second, the capacity of the muscles to burn fat increases, due to increased activity of the aerobic machinery within the muscles.

If you want to increase your capacity for fat utilization, make sure your workouts last at least an hour. The longer, the better. Also, keep your intensity low. If your workout is too intensive (over 70% of aerobic capacity), you may produce lactic acid, which will suppress your fat mobilization. Your muscles will then shift from using fat to using glycogen more as fuel.

High intensity workouts, (e.g., with interval training) are done to increase speed, not to improve fat utilization. (You may also increase the availability of fat by consuming caffeine prior to exercise. We'll discuss the pros and cons of caffeine in Chapter 11.)

Your aerobic capacity and anaerobic threshold will also affect the contribution of fat during endurance exercise. In general, the higher your aerobic capacity and anaerobic threshold, the greater your ability to use fat.

Fat Loading

Until recently, nutritional strategies for preparing for endurance exercise assumed that endurance can only be improved by either increasing muscle glycogen stores or slowing down their rate of utilization by ingesting caffeine prior to exercise. However, a popularized study of the value of high-fat diets has led some endurance athletes to try "fat loading" in place of carbohydrate loading.

This study* evaluated how a high-fat diet affected cycling time to exhaustion and muscle glycogen utilization. The subjects ate an average American diet and then exercised to exhaustion at 63% of $\dot{V}O_{2max}$. Later they ate a high-fat diet (85% of calories), which was low in carbohydrate (less than 80 calories of carbohydrate per day). After four weeks on this diet, they again exercised to exhaustion at 63% of $\dot{V}O_{2max}$.

The exercise time to exhaustion was not significantly different on the two diets (147 minutes and 152 minutes respectively). But after adapting to the high-fat diet, muscle glycogen utilization dropped four-fold and glucose utilization dropped three-fold on the bike ride to exhaustion. Fat utilization increased to make up the difference.

Don't buy that steak yet, though. The drawbacks of high-fat diets outweigh any potential benefits. Such diets need medical supervision; they have been associated with sudden death and heart rhythm disturbances, due to loss of protein from the heart and potassium depletion. Since exercise by itself does not fully protect against heart disease, eating a high-fat diet for a prolonged period may contribute to an increased risk of developing heart disease.

Metabolism, 32:769-776, 1983

The cyclists in the study were constantly monitored for electrolyte losses and these were replaced throughout the experiment. Also, although the cyclists trained heavily, their blood cholesterol levels increased while on the high-fat diets.

A high-fat diet is also hard to digest. The high-fat meals in this study consisted of butter, cheese, cream, ground or marbled beef and tuna with dollups of mayonnaise. Such diets tend to become unappetizing after a bit; also, they lack the variety needed to meet general nutritional requirements.

Adapting to a high-fat diet takes at least two weeks. Exercising during this time will be difficult and unpleasant, due to low glycogen stores. Even when adaptation is complete, the ability to exercise hard (75% or more of $\dot{V}O_{2max}$) may be impaired. Keep in mind that in many events you're competing at 75% or more of your $\dot{V}O_{2max}$.

In addition, the study can be faulted because it did not compare a high-carbohydrate diet (70% of calories) to the high-fat diet. A high-carbohydrate diet would provide higher glycogen stores and thus result in a longer cycling time to exhaustion than the 50% carbohydrate diet used in the study.

Also, the cyclists exercised to exhaustion at an exercise intensity low enough (63% of $\dot{V}O_{2max}$) to be fueled by fat and not limited by muscle glycogen depletion. If these tests had been conducted at an exercise intensity known to be limited by muscle glycogen depletion (75% or more of $\dot{V}O_{2max}$), impaired endurance would have been probable.

So a high-fat diet may not buy you any endurance advantage after all. And why feel lousy for four weeks while you're trying to adjust to a high-fat diet when you can feel good and perform well (without any adaptation) on a high-carbohydrate diet?

In any case, the potential adverse health effects make high-fat diets too risky for endurance training.

Chapter 7

Protein
The Great American
Protein Myth

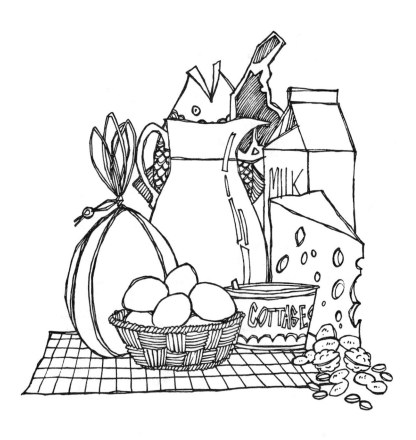

A friend of mine in her late twenties had been running for ten years. She felt good during runs, but felt she needed to lose weight, so she went on a diet.

While on the diet, she complained that she had no energy, to the point where at times, she couldn't run at all. "What's the diet?" I asked her.

For breakfast she had an egg; at lunch, a protein supplement with milk; and for dinner she ate cottage cheese, a hamburger patty and a piece of bread.

I asked her what she really wanted to eat. "Sweets," she said, "I want sweets."

I told her to come off the diet and eat more bread, fruits and vegetables and starchy foods in general. She kept the level of calories she was eating the same. She lost her craving for sweets, had plenty of energy and felt fine.

If this woman couldn't find the energy to run, she must have felt very bad. She later told me that it had been easier to run while pregnant than it had been to run on that diet.

She was eating so much protein that she couldn't maintain her glycogen stores. She didn't get enough carbohydrates to perform well.

Americans have been sold on the idea that proteins are the good guys. In fact they are essential, for general health and body maintenance, and vigorous exercise makes some special demands on protein supplies. But proteins are no "more essential" than other needed nutrients. They are a poor energy source, and too much can be detrimental, as well as expensive. And a balanced diet supplies more than enough for any athlete.

Protein in the Diet

Protein is a major structural component of all body tissue and is needed for growth and repair. Proteins are also necessary components of hormones, enzymes and blood plasma transport systems.

Protein is widely distributed in plant and animal foods. Good sources of protein include beef, pork, chicken, fish, dairy products, split peas and beans. A well-balanced vegetarian diet can easily supply enough protein, because protein is found in so many plant foods. Adequate vegetarian diets can be particularly healthy, because they're usually lower in fat and higher in complex carbohydrates than the average American diet.

The proteins in both plant and animal sources are composed of the same basic structural units — amino acids. Some plant foods are short particular amino acids, and must be paired with other foods that supply those that are lacking. Amino acids from different plant foods can be paired (e.g., beans and rice) to complement each other and provide the variety that is needed for effective protein function.

Protein Needs and Exercise

Current research on protein requirements during training suggests that athletes need more protein than sedentary people. Exercise may promote a loss of muscle protein through reduced protein synthesis and increased protein breakdown. The hormonal changes which occur during exercise — decreased insulin and increased epinephrine (adrenalin) — may be responsible for these effects of exercise on protein metabolism.

Exercise may also promote body protein metabolism, and promote body protein loss in other ways — it has been found in the urine of runners after marathons, and may also be lost in sweat.

On the other hand, regular physical training tends to reduce muscle protein breakdown and protein loss from the body. Although protein breakdown may predominate during exercise, protein synthesis is enhanced in the recovery period that follows. Regular exercise appears to increase the efficiency of this protein synthesis during recovery.

The net long-term effect of regular exercise is through protein build-up. Because of this, and because Americans in general ingest far more protein than they can use, an athlete on a sound balanced diet should not seek sources of additional protein.

Protein as Fuel

As I've described, a number of different factors influence the particular fuel used during exercise. The two factors which appear to influence the use of protein the most are the duration of exercise and the carbohydrate content of the diet. When muscle glycogen stores are low, as the result either of prolonged exercise or a low-carbohydrate diet, protein may contribute as much as 10% of the energy for exercise. On the other hand, when muscle glyocogen stores are high, the contribution of protein for energy is no more than about 5%. (You will also use more protein for fuel when your total caloric intake is inadequate, as during fasting or semi-starvation.) Thus, by maintaining muscle glycogen stores, a high-carbohydrate diet during training helps reduce the use of protein as a fuel.

Protein and Glucose

Your body relies on the carbohydrate in food to keep your blood glucose (sugar) at the constant level needed to maintain proper functioning of your central nervous system. If you don't eat enough carbohydrate, your liver glycogen is broken down to supply glucose for the blood. After liver glycogen is depleted, the most readily available source of glucose is protein. The body actually begins to use its protein stores to obtain this vital sugar.

How Much Protein

The recommended dietary allowance (RDA) of protein for sedentary adults is .8 grams per kilogram of body weight. Current research[*] suggests that endurance athletes need 1.2 gram per kilogram and may benefit by consuming up to 2 grams per kilogram, during periods of prolonged heavy endurance exercise.

An increased protein intake appears to be more important during the early stages of training than later in the training program. In the early stages, you require more protein to support increases in your muscle mass, red blood cell formation, myoglobin (an oxygen carrier in the muscle similar to hemoglobin), and aerobic enzymes in the muscle.

[*]*Med Sci Sports Excer*, 19:S179-S190,1987

Protein in the Food You Eat

Although you do need more if you're an endurance athlete, you still can easily obtain enough protein through your diet. The average American consumes about 100 grams of protein per day (70% from foods which singly contain all the necessary amino acids), with a total protein intake averaging about 1.4 grams per kilogram. Exercising increases your caloric needs, and accordingly your average protein intake.

For example, let's say that a sedentary 70-kilogram man decides to train for a marathon. Over a period of time, his daily caloric intake gradually increases from 2,500 to 5,000 calories. His protein intake would increase from 75 to 150 grams per day if 12% of his calories came from protein. His protein intake by weight would increase from 1.1 to 2.1 grams per kilogram, which would be ample.

Protein/Amino Acid Supplements

If you eat a reasonably balanced diet, you do not need protein (or amino acid) supplements, because your diet already provides enough protein for growth and repair. Extra protein doesn't help and may hurt. Protein supplements are ineffective in promoting endurance and/or increasing muscle mass.

Your body can't distinguish between the protein you obtain from food and costly protein or amino acid supplements. When you eat more protein than you require, you will use it for energy or convert it to fat. Protein is expensive; carbohydrate provides energy more efficiently, and at less cost.

Some athletes take free-amino acid supplements, supposedly to enhance their performance. Proponents of these supplements claim that they are more readily digested and absorbed than the protein from food. There are also claims that certain amino acids increase muscle mass and decrease body fat.

The claims made for free-amino acid supplements aren't valid. Free-amino acid proponents claim that only a small amount of the amino acids in food are digested and absorbed — in fact, 85 to 99% of the protein from animal sources and about 90% of the protein from vegetable sources is absorbed and utilized.

Proponents also claim that since free-amino acids do not need to be digested before absorption, they replenish the body's proteins faster. There is no evidence that more rapid absorption is benefical — it takes hours, not minutes to rebuild muscle proteins damaged during intense exercise.

There is the further claim for the supplements that they are less taxing on the digestive system. Actually, the body quite readily produces an array of digestive enzymes that systematically break down the protein in food to free-amino acids, which are then absorbed. (Thus, chicken or beans are in fact a "time release" source of amino acids.) Amino acid supplements usually only provide 200 to 500 milligrams of amino acids per capsule. One ounce of beef, chicken, or fish provides 7 grams of protein — 7,000 milligrams of amino acids!

One thing is clear: free-amino acid supplements contain no other nutrients. Thus their use in lieu of protein-rich foods invites deficiencies of other nutrients (e.g., niacin, thiamine and iron) provided by those foods.

Excess amino acids from whatever source, which cannot be incorporated into new proteins, are either used for energy, or else converted to fat. When this happens, excess urea is produced, which increases the body's need for water (and thus invites dehydration).

Arginine and ornithine are particularly popular as supplements since they supposedly stimulate the secretion of growth hormone — in theory resulting in increased muscle mass and decreased body fat. There's no evidence that the amount of amino acids provided by supplements has any effect on growth hormone levels or body composition. Exercise by itself increases growth hormone levels significantly.

There may be as yet unidentified long-term risks associated with amino acid supplementation. But in any event, it makes no sense to take a supplement that has not been proven safe or effective — particularly when that product is promoted primarily by people who stand to gain financially.

High-Protein Diets

High-protein diets are also generally high in fat. This type of diet is poor for maintaining muscle glycogen stores — a high-protein, high-fat diet consumed after strenuous exercise will produce slow or incomplete replacement of muscle glycogen.

Protein also takes a long time to digest, whereas carbohydrates are rapidly digested. And consuming too much protein (whether through food or supplements) increases your body's water requirement, and may contribute to dehydration. This is because your kidneys need more water to eliminate the extra nitrogen load imposed by the excess protein.

As you can see, the current fascination with protein/ amino acid supplementation is at best wasteful, and can actually hurt your athletic performance.

Chapter 8

Vitamins and Minerals

Is More Better?

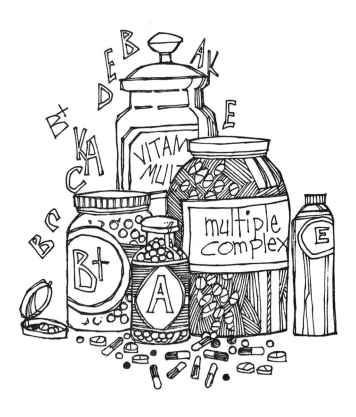

I was working with an athlete who was taking loads of vitamins.

"Is it all right to take all these vitamins?" he asked me.

I told him about the possible hazards of taking megadoses, then asked: "Do you notice any difference?"

The only thing he'd noticed was that his urine was very yellow.

"What about your performance? Are you doing any better?" I asked him.

"I hope so," he said. "I've spent so much money on vitamins that I'd like to think they're doing something."

Many people take massive doses of vitamin/mineral supplements which far exceed their needs. They are assuming that if a small amount of nutrient is good, more will be better. In addition to seeking a competitive edge, they sometimes feel that their diets are inadequate — and take supplements for "nutritional insurance."

In general, vitamin/mineral supplements are unnecessary, if you get a sound, well-balanced diet. But two minerals, calcium and iron, are often in short supply in the American diet, and are worth special consideration — with the advice of a health professional.

Vitamins

Vitamins are organic molecules, which the body cannot manufacture but requires in small amounts. They are metabolic regulators which govern the processes of energy production, growth, maintenance and repair. Currently, 13 vitamins have been identified — each with a special function (though vitamins also work in complicated ways with other nutrients).

Contrary to popular belief, vitamins do not provide a direct source of energy. This means that in general the vitamin requirements of an athlete are not significantly greater than those of a sedentary person.

Thiamine is an exception, because it is required in proportion to calories consumed and active people need more calories. But a sound diet provides ample thiamine. It is supplied by those carbohydrate-rich foods recommended for athletes — breads and other whole grain or fortified grain products.

Water-Soluble/Fat-Soluble

Vitamins are divided into two groups — water-soluble and fat-soluble. A, D, E and K are soluble in fat, whereas C and the B vitamins are soluble in water. The solubility characteristic is important in determining whether the body can store the vitamin or whether the supply must be constantly replenished.

When the intake of water-soluble vitamins is greater than you require, the excess is excreted. Although this is a great way to increase the vitamin content of your urine, it doesn't help your performance. Fat-soluble vitamins cannot be excreted and are instead stored in body fat, principally in the liver. Over a long time (or not so long if vitamin supplements are taken), this build-up of fat-soluble vitamins can produce serious toxic effects, particularly through the accumulation of vitamins A and D.

More is Not Better

The National Academy of Sciences has established (and regularly reconsiders) recommended dietary allowances (RDA's) as a guide for determining nutritional needs. (See the Appendix.) Simply, the RDA is the daily amount of a nutrient recommended for practically all healthy individuals to promote optimal health. It is not a minimal amount needed to prevent disease symptoms — a large margin of safety is figured in. For example, the body needs approximately 10 milligrams of vitamin C to prevent the deficiency disease scurvy, but the RDA is set at 60 milligrams.

In general, the nutrient needs for the average person are only about two-thirds of the RDA. This means that as long as athletes consume at least 67% of the RDA for a given nutrient, they are generally protected from a nutritional deficiency.

Megadoses of vitamins and minerals (amounts at least 10 times the RDA) can be dangerous. When vitamins are taken in such amounts they no longer function as vitamins — they function as drugs, often producing the same serious side effects.

As mentioned earlier, fat-soluble vitamins in particular may build up in the body to toxic levels. But excessive intake of water-soluble vitamins may also pose problems. Large amounts of niacin, for example, can induce burning or tingling of the skin, rash, nausea and diarrhea. High doses of niacin also interfere with fat mobilization and speed up glycogen depletion.

Minerals

Minerals serve a variety of functions in the body. Some are used to build tissue, such as calcium and phosphorus for bones and teeth. Others are important components of hormones, such as iodine in thyroxine. Iron is crucial in the formation of hemoglobin — the oxygen carrier within red blood cells.

Minerals are also significant for a number of regulatory functions. These include regulation of muscle contraction, conduction of nerve impulses and regulation of normal heart rhythm.

Minerals are classified into two groups, based upon the amounts the body needs. Major minerals, such as calcium, are those needed in the diet at levels greater than 100 milligrams a day. Minor minerals (trace elements) such as iron, are those where fewer than 100 milligrams a day are required. Calcium and iron are both minerals of special concern for endurance athletes, particularly women.

Calcium

Calcium is the most abundant mineral in the body. The bones and teeth contain 99% of the body's calcium. The other 1% circulates in the blood, serving several vital functions. Calcium is critical for the conduction of nerve impulses, heart function, muscle contraction and the operation of certain enzymes.

The bones act as a calcium reservoir if the supply of calcium in the blood runs too low. Your body has an elaborate system in which hormones interact to keep the calcium level in the blood within a narrow range. This means that despite what you have heard, when you have muscle cramps, they aren't due to a calcium deficiency.

The RDA for calcium is 800 milligrams per day for adult men and women age 25 and up. However, the National Institute of Health (NIH), along with many nutrition experts, recommends that post-menopausal women increase their calcium intake, to reduce the incidence of osteoporosis. The NIH also recommends a higher calcium intake for men to prevent bone loss as they age. The typical American diet supplies a meager 450 to 550 milligrams a day, and most people need to consume more calcium.

The current RDA for adolescent women is 1,200 milligrams per day. Pre-menopausal adult women should consume 1,000 milligrams per day. Women of any age who are on estrogen replacement therapy should also consume 1,000 milligrams per day, because they can still lose bone mass. Post-menopausal women who aren't on estrogen should consume 1,500 milligrams per day.

Osteoporosis. Osteoporosis is an age-related disorder in which bone mass decreases and the susceptibility to fractures increases. It is a major public health problem in our country. Osteoporosis is called the "silent disease" because it usually goes undetected until a fracture occurs — the most common being of the hip, wrist or spine. The most effective method of detection (bone loss as slight as 1%) is called densitometry; it is available in several medical centers.

Figure 10
Sources of Calcium

All quantities are one cup unless indicated otherwise. Some good sources of calcium are also high in sodium, indicated with an asterisk (*). If you are not restricting sodium too much, you can still include these in your diet.

Milk & Dairy Products	mg	Nuts, Legumes	mg
Milk, nonfat	300	Almonds, ½ cup	173
Low-fat fruit-flavored yogurt	345	Lentils, cooked	50
Low-fat plain yogurt	415	Dried beans, cooked	90
*Cottage cheese, 2%	155	**Vegetables**	
*Cheddar cheese, 1 oz.	204	Certain leafy green	280
*Mozzarella, part skim, 1 oz.	183	vegetables, including dandelion greens,	
*Parmesan, 1 oz.	390	mustard greens, tur-	
Ricotta, part skim, 1 oz.	77	nip greens, collards	
*Swiss, 1 oz.	272	and kale, but *exclud-*	
Tofu, 3½ oz.	127	*ing* spinach, beet greens, and chard	

Fish		Water	
*Salmon, canned, 3 oz.	167	"Hard" water, 1 qt.	100
*Sardines, canned, 3 oz.	326	"Soft" water, 1 qt.	30

Source: *Maximize Your Body Potential*, by Joyce D. Nash, PhD, Bull Publishing Company, Palo Alto, CA. Used with permission.

Exercise enhances skeletal calcium absorption, thus exerting a protective effect against osteoporosis. The benefits of exercise in increasing bone mass have been demonstrated with both young and elderly men and women. Weight bearing aerobic exercise is ideal for helping to prevent osteoporosis, as well as heart disease.

Estrogen loss, along with an inadequate calcium intake, are considered the main causes of osteoporosis. Women are more susceptible to osteoporosis than men because of their lesser bone mass, and menopause related decline in estrogen. In addition to consuming a calcium-rich diet and exercising, not smoking and moderating caffeine and alcohol intake will decrease the risk of developing osteoporosis.

Amenorrhea. Some women who exercise strenuously stop menstruating — a condition called athletic amenorrhea. Although the specific cause of athletic amenorrhea is unknown and may vary among women, it appears to coincide with decreased estrogen production. Since estrogen deficiency is an important risk factor for the development of osteoporosis, amenorrhea may predispose female athletes to early onset osteoporosis and fractures. Spinal bone mass has been found to be lower in amenorrheic women runners.*

However, it is not recommended that amenorrheic women athletes stop exercising. In fact, exercise may partially overcome the calcium withdrawal from the skeleton associated with estrogen deficiency. But women with athletic amenorrhea should consult a physician to rule out any serious medical problems, and all amenorrheic women should maintain a calcium intake of 1,500 milligrams per day. After consultation with a physician, any or all of the following may be recommended: estrogen replacement therapy, weight gain, diet modification, and reduced training.

Calcium in the Diet. How can you get enough calcium from your diet? Dairy products are the best general source, since all are high in calcium and their calcium has a high rate of absorption. An eight-ounce glass of milk or a ⅓

*N Engl J Med, 311: 277-281, 1984.

cup of powdered non-fat milk each contains about 300 milligrams of calcium. Skim or low-fat versions of milk, cheese, yogurt and cottage cheese are excellent reduced-fat (and reduced calorie) sources of calcium.

Other good sources of calcium are sardines (because of the bones) and oysters. Broccoli and greens (kale, collard, turnip and mustard) are good sources of calcium without any fat. Tofu which has been processed with calcium sulfate also can be a good source of calcium.

Supplements.   Should calcium supplements be used? Before taking a supplement, consult a registered dietitian or physician for advice on how to obtain the appropriate amounts respectively from food and, if appropriate from supplements.

Calcium intake should not exceed recommended levels because of the risk of urinary tract stones for susceptible people.

Calcium carbonate (Tums® or a generic equivalent) is an inexpensive and acceptable calcium source. Such antacids that contain calcium are practically the same as dietary supplements. The primary difference between the two is in the marketing — when calcium carbonate is sold as a calcium supplement, it costs more.

Bone meal and dolomite should not be used as calcium supplements because they may contain harmful amounts of lead, arsenic, mercury and other potentially toxic minerals.

Iron

Iron deserves special attention because of the prevalence of iron deficiency anemia — characterized by a low hemoglobin level (hemoglobin values below 12 mg/dl for women and 14 mg/dl for men are considered anemic). Women, in comparison to men, are much more likely to suffer from iron deficiency anemia. Iron deficiency in women is usually the result of menstrual blood losses, together with inadequate dietary intake.

As I said, iron is necessary for the formation of hemoglobin. When the total hemoglobin concentration drops due to anemia, the muscles don't receive as much oxygen. An anemic person has less endurance and can't exercise as hard because her aerobic capacity is reduced.

Iron and the Athlete. Exercise may cause iron loss, and increase the risk of developing iron deficiency for both men and women. Results of recent studies suggest that exercise causes accelerated destruction of red blood cells, possibly due to mechanical trauma (e.g., hitting the ground while running) and gastrointestinal bleeding.

Normally, iron absorption increases when iron intake is inadequate. However, iron-deficient athletes have been found to have one-half the absorption rates of iron-deficient sedentary people.* Exercise also causes an increased iron loss in the sweat.

The message is clear: male and female endurance athletes must take special care to consume the RDA for iron — 15 milligrams for women, 10 milligrams for men. The average American diet supplies only 5 to 6 milligrams of iron per 1,000 calories. Women athletes typically consume 10 milligrams of iron per day — far less than the RDA.

Iron in the Diet. How can you obtain enough iron? Animal sources should be emphasized, since iron from them is absorbed better than iron from vegetable sources. Combining animal and vegetable products (e.g., meat and bean burrito) increases the iron absorbed from the vegetable product. Vitamin C also enhances iron absorption, so high vitamin C foods (e.g., orange juice) should be consumed in conjunction with foods containing iron (like cream of wheat) for optimum absorption.

* *Med Sci Sports Exer,* 12:61-64, 1980

Figure 11
Sources of Iron

Food	Measuring Unit	Iron (mg.)
*Liver-pork	3 oz.	17.7
*Liver-lamb	3 oz.	12.6
*Liver-chicken	3 oz.	8.4
*Liver-beef	3 oz.	6.6
*Oysters, fried	3 oz.	5.9
Tostada, bean	1	3.2
Dried apricots	½ cup (12 halves)	3.0
Baked beans with pork and molasses	½ cup	3.0
Soybeans, cooked	½ cup	2.7
*Beef	3 oz.	2.7
*Beef enchilada	1	2.6
Raisins	½ cup	2.5
Lima beans, canned or fresh cooked	½ cup	2.5
Refried beans	½ cup	2.3
Dried figs	½ cup (4 figs)	2.2
Spinach, cooked	½ cup	2.0
*Taco-beef	1	2.0
Mustard greens, cooked	½ cup	1.8
Corn tortilla, lime treated	8" diameter	1.6
Prune juice	½ cup	1.5
Peas, fresh cooked	½ cup	1.4
Enchilada, cheese and sour cream	1	1.4
Egg	1 large	1.2
*Turkey, roasted	3 oz.	1.1
Sardines, canned in oil	1 oz (2 medium)	1.0

*Foods of animal origin. Iron in foods of animal origin (except milk, which has little iron) is absorbed twice as efficiently as iron in foods of plant origin.

Source: *Food for Sport*, by Nathan J. Smith, MD and Bonnie Worthington-Roberts, PhD, 1989. Bull Publishing Company, Palo Alto, CA. Used with permission.

Cast iron cookware also increases the iron content of foods. The more acidic and the longer the food is cooked, the higher the residual iron content of the food.

Red meat is an excellent iron source — containing about 1 milligram of iron per ounce. Iron-enriched or fortified cereal/grain products can contribute significantly, and peas, split peas, beans and some dark vegetables are good vegetable sources of iron.

Iron Deficiency. Those at risk for iron deficiency, particularly menstruating women athletes, should have their hemoglobin level checked routinely. A more expensive, but more sensitive test for iron deficiency measures serum ferritin (storage iron). Low ferritin levels appear in the first stage of iron deficiency, representing inadequate iron stores in your bone marrow. The test is valuable because it detects iron deficiency early before hemoglobin drops to anemic levels.

A low ferritin level means that you have an increased risk for developing iron deficiency anemia. You can increase your stores through a high-iron diet and head off the consequences of anemia.

Iron Supplements. It is a challenge to get 15 milligrams of iron a day from food — so shouldn't women take iron supplements? Perhaps, but you should have good advice. A high iron intake can produce an iron overload and cause deficiencies of other trace minerals (e.g., zinc and copper). Iron supplementation will not improve your health or performance if you have normal iron stores.

As with calcium, it is wise to consult a registered dietitian or physician before taking a supplement. If supplements are used, they should not exceed the RDA, unless medically indicated and prescribed by a physician.

Supplements

The Council on Scientific Affairs of the American Medical Association has published a report on the appropriate use of vitamin supplements. Healthy adult men and women who aren't pregnant or breastfeeding do not require vitamin supplements — provided they're eating a balanced and varied diet.

The Council concedes that, due to changing dietary habits (increased consumption of processed foods and of meals away from home), there may be instances where vitamin intake is inadequate. Before opting for supplementation, however, an attempt should be made to improve food selection and eating habits. When a supplement is chosen, the dose should not exceed 150% of the RDA.

Supplements containing two to ten times the RDA of any vitamin should be considered therapeutic and used only under medical supervision. In such cases, the supplement is used to treat specific disease states or conditions that limit absorption or utilization of a specific vitamin or increase the requirement for it.

The AMA Council condemns the increasing use of megadose therapy because it is based on anecdotal, non-scientific evidence. Megadose therapy only thins pocketbooks and builds false hopes, without providing any beneficial results. More important, the consumption of large amounts of vitamins and minerals can produce toxic effects and/or impair the delicate metabolic interaction among vital nutrients.

Nutrition quacks have invented the perfect diseases to insure their income — "subclinical illnesses." These are medical problems which supposedly plague almost everyone, yet cannot be detected by standard medical tests. Quacks exploit athletes by insisting that their "run down feeling" is due to a vitamin or mineral deficiency. In fact, when there is a nutritional reason for fatigue, it is usually a lack of calories or carbohydrate.

The athlete with fatigue could be fasting, crash dieting, eating too little carbohydrate for adequate glycogen synthesis, or over-training. When people feel better after taking supplements, it's due to the strength of their belief that supplements help — the placebo effect. (It's cheaper, and often healthier, to believe in food.)

As a general proposition, megavitamin therapy is an inappropriate form of self-medication — you can obtain enough vitamins and minerals from your diet. Supplements at levels exceeding the RDA do not improve the performance of a well-nourished athlete.

Undernourished Athletes

True, vitamin and mineral deficiencies can impair performance, but it is unusual for athletes to have such deficiencies. They eat more than sedentary people and so tend to get more vitamins and minerals in relation to their needs.

Athletes who limit their caloric intake, however, are at risk for nutritional deficiencies — those concerned about how extra weight affects performance, or about cosmetics, who increase exercise while limiting food intake may be at nutritional risk. Often these are athletes competing in long distance running, gymnastics, figure skating and diving, and those required to "make weight" — wrestlers, boxers, and weight classified football or crew participants. Weight conscious casual athletes may also be at risk.

A vitamin/mineral supplement supplying 100% of the RDA might be appropriate for these individuals.

Taking the Easy Way

It's much easier to take vitamin/mineral supplements than to change the way you eat. Supplements provide the illusion of caring for your health, but remove the burden of dietary change. You can't do it just with a pill. Just as an adequate diet is not enhanced by supplementation, an inadequate diet is not redeemed by supplementation.

By eating a variety of high quality foods from each of the exchange lists each day, you eliminate the need for vitamin/mineral supplementation. To improve your "nutritional insurance," you can also eat more complex carbohydrates and less "empty calories" (sugar, fat and alcohol).

Chapter 9

Hydration
Don't Forget to Drink

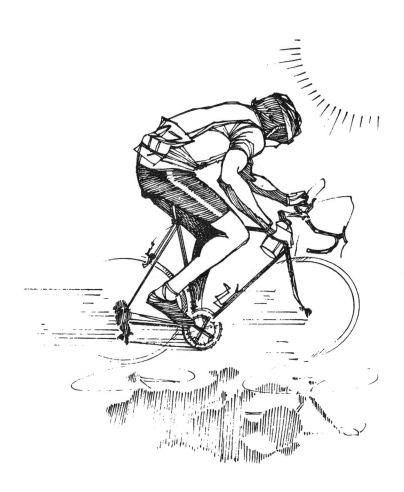

I was the second person to get into lunch at the 100-mile mark of a 200-mile ride. It was 100 degrees and I was tired.

I started the second 100 miles with two full water bottles. No shade. Hilly steep pitches. I was going very slowly and still felt terrible, riding in my lowest gear. Ten miles out I had gone through both water bottles.

There was no escape from the heat. Cycling produced more heat. Raging thirst. I searched for water but the hills were parched. I felt they would find my bleached bones on the side of the road.

I became disoriented and was on the verge of crying. Not thinking clearly, I went on for 30 more miles. Rounding a corner I thought I saw a bicyclist in need of help and stopped. There was no one there. I was hallucinating. I stopped.

Other experienced riders felt the same thing — throbbing heads, hot/cold flashes, and sudden weakness. Only 20% of those who started the race finished. The environment was so harsh that we couldn't drink enough fluids to replace our losses.

With all the concern about various nutrients, and all the dollars spent in pursuit of the competitive edge, it is amazing how often athletes ignore the importance of fluids. They can easily ruin their performance, and endanger their health, when they fail to maintain adequate fluid levels.

Water is the most essential of all nutrients, since your body requires it constantly. An adequate supply of water is essential for all energy production in the body, for temperature control (particularly during exercise), and for elimination of waste products from metabolism. Dehydration reduces endurance and increases the risk of heat illnesses (heat exhaustion and heat stroke).

Hydration and Exercise

Water is the most commonly overlooked endurance aid. Adequate hydration is essential for optimum performance. When the air temperature exceeds the core (deep body) and skin temperatures, you must rely primarily on the evaporation of sweat to dissipate heat. The loss of body fluids in sweat gradually compromises your ability to circulate blood and regulate body temperature.

During exercise in the heat, blood that was transferring oxygen to the muscles is diverted to the skin to transfer heat from the body's core to the environment. This competition for blood between muscles and skin places a greater demand on the cardiovascular system. Consequently, as you become dehydrated, your heart rate increases, the blood flow to your skin begins to decrease

and your temperature rises steadily to the danger zone —
105 to 106 degrees F.

In practical terms, your performance begins to decline
and maintaining a steady level of exercise intensity
becomes more difficult. During prolonged exercise in the
heat, sweat losses constituting as little as 2% of your body
weight will impair circulatory and heat regulatory functions. (Long distance runners can have sweat losses of up
to 6 to 10% of their total weight.)

Inadequate fluid intake speeds up dehydration, and can
ultimately result in a serious, indeed life-threatening health
problem.

Besides heat, relative humidity is also important. As the
moisture in the air increases, the effectiveness of evaporation through sweating decreases. If the air is saturated
with water, little evaporation will occur even at cooler
temperatures. Sweating helps to cool your body, but only
if the sweat evaporates from the skin. So beware of intense
physical exertion, not only on hot days, but also on warm,
humid days.

If you wear a sweat suit, there is no opportunity for
evaporation. People who exercise in sweat suits (or worse,
full rubber suits during hot weather) to lose weight or just
"to get in shape," endanger their health and even their
lives. (And any extra weight loss is just water, which must
be replaced.)

Maintaining Hydration

You can prepare for exercise in hot weather by drinking
14 to 20 ounces of cold fluid 10 to 15 minutes before
exercise. This technique, known as *hyper-hydration*, helps
to lower your body's core temperature and thus to reduce
the added stress heat places on the cardiovascular system.

Figure 12
Schematic Diagram Showing Heat Production Within
Working Skeletal Muscle, its Transport to the Body Core
and to the Skin, and its Subsequent Exchange
with the Environment

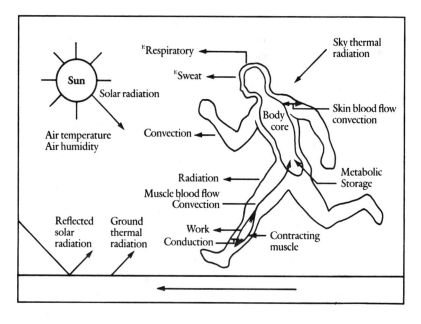

Source: Reprinted with permission of Macmillan Publishing Company from *Exercise and Sport Scientist Reviews*, Vol. 12 by V. C. Gisolfi, C. G. Wenger. Copyright 1984 by American College of Sports Medicine.

During exercise, you should drink 3 to 6 ounces of fluid every 10 to 15 minutes to replace sweat losses and maintain blood volume. Although larger volumes empty more rapidly from the stomach, most athletes are uncomfortable exercising with a nearly full stomach.

Cold drinks empty more rapidly from the stomach than warm drinks. Reducing the temperature of the stomach increases the flow of fluids from the stomach into the intestine. Cold drinks don't harm the heart, and contrary to popular belief, they do not cause cramping. Inadequate intake is the primary obstacle to fluid replacement. Thirst is not an adequate guide, and it is important to regulate fluid replacement by drinking fluids according to a schedule, rather than in response to thirst. Get in the habit of regular drinking during training. Many athletes only drink during competition. Heat injury can occur just as easily during training. Adequate fluid consumption during training not only protects against heat injury but gives you the chance to practice proper hydration techniques.

Be aware of the signs and symptoms associated with heat illness. These include unusual fatigue, weakness, irritability, dizziness, disorientation and nausea.

Weigh yourself before and after exercise (nude is best) to determine how much water you're losing. Drink 2 cups of fluid for every pound of weight lost. If you notice a gradual loss of weight during hot weather training, it may be due to chronic dehydration rather than fat loss.

Choice of Fluid

Should you drink water or a sports drink? Extensive research has been done on fluid replacement beverages.

Early studies* suggested that drinks containing more than 2.5% carbohydrate left the stomach more slowly than water. Unfortunately, these studies focused on the stomach and ignored the intestines. As a result, it became widely believed that sports drinks aren't absorbed rapidly and therefore compromise body temperature regulation and performance.

This belief is unfounded. A sports drink may leave the stomach more slowly than water because of its higher

* *J Appl Physiol*, 37:679-683, 1974

caloric content, but once it reaches the intestine, it is absorbed more rapidly. The sugar and sodium found in sports drinks actually enhance fluid absorption in the small intestine.

Sports drinks are absorbed as well as water, and in events of moderate duration, they provide greater performance benefits. Recent research** suggests that a 6% carbohydrate solution enters the blood as rapidly as water. Both drinks had the same favorable influence on temperature regulation, cardiovascular function, and fluid replacement. But only the sugar solution improved endurance by providing energy to exercising muscles.

For optimal absorption and performance, a sports drink should contain 6 to 8% carbohydrate. It is doubtful that drinks containing less carbohydrate will help endurance. Those that exceed 10% carbohydrate (fruit juices, sodas, and concentrated fructose drinks) will take longer to be absorbed and may cause abdominal cramps, nausea, bloating, and diarrhea.***

Several sports drinks use glucose polymers (maltodextrins) as their carbohydrate source. Maltodextrins are created by breaking down corn starch into small glucose chains (polymers). The companies that make these drinks claim these liquids will be more rapidly absorbed than sports drinks containing glucose. They aren't. A recent study**** compared consumption of a 10% glucose drink and 10% glucose polymer drink during prolonged (two hour) treadmill running in the heat and neither drink performed significantly better than the other.

Electrolytes

Electrolytes (sodium, chloride, and potassium) are necessary for the maintenance of fluid levels and muscle

**Am J Clin Nutr*, 48:1023-1030, 1988
****Sports Med*, 3:247-274, 1986
*****Med Sci Sports Exerc*, 18:568-575, 1986

Figure 13
Fluid Replacement Beverage Comparison Chart

Beverage	Flavors	Carbohydrate Ingredient	Carbohydrate Concentration (percent)	Sodium (milligrams) per 8 oz. serving	Potassium (milligrams) per 8 oz. serving	Other Minerals and Vitamins
GATORADE® Thirst Quencher The Quaker Oats Company	Lemon-Lime, Lemonade, Fruit Punch, Orange, Citrus Cooler	Powder: Sucrose/ Glucose Liquid: Sucrose/ Glucose Syrup Solids	6	110	25	Chloride, Phosphorus
GATORADE® Light	Lemon-Lime, Orange, Citrus Cooler	Glucose	2.5	80	25	Trace
Quickick® Cramer Products, Inc.	Lemon-Lime, Fruit Punch, Orange, Grape, Lemonade	Fructose/Sucrose	4.7	116	23	Calcium, Chloride, Phosphorus
Sqwincher® The Activity Drink Universal Products, Inc.	Lemon-Lime, Fruit Punch, Lemonade, Orange, Grape, Strawberry, Grapefruit	Glucose/Fructose	6.8	60	36	Vitamin C, Chloride, Phosphorus, Calcium, Magnesium
Exceed® Ross Laboratories	Lemon-Lime, Orange	Glucose Polymers/ Fructose	7.2	50	45	Calcium, Magnesium, Phosphorus, Chloride
PowerBurst™ PowerBurst Corp.	Orange, Lemon-Lime, Lemonade, Berry Punch	Fructose	6.0	35	55	Vitamin C, A, E, Chloride, Magnesium, Calcium, B-vitamins, Pantothenic Acid, Folic Acid, Biotin

Figure 13 (continued)
Fluid Replacement Beverage Comparison Chart

Beverage	Flavors	Carbohydrate Ingredient	Carbohydrate Concentration (percent)	Sodium (milligrams) per 8 oz. serving	Potassium (milligrams) per 8 oz. serving	Other Minerals and Vitamins
Body Fuel® 450 Vitex Foods, Inc.	Orange	Maltodextrin, Fructose	4.2	80	20	Phosphorus, Chloride, Iron, Vitamins A, C, B-vitamins
10-K® Beverage Products, Inc.	Lemon-Lime, Orange, Fruit Punch, Lemonade, Iced Tea	Sucrose, Glucose, Fructose	6.3	52	26	Vitamin C, Chloride, Phosphorus
Mountain Dew® Sport Pepsico, Inc.	Regular	High Fructose Corn Syrup/Sucrose	10	60	40	Vitamin C, Chloride, Calcium
	Diet	none	0	40	45	Vitamin C, Chloride, Calcium
Soft Drinks	Cola, Non-cola	High Fructose Corn Syrup/Sucrose	10.2-11.3	9.2-28	Trace	Phosphorus
Diet Soft Drinks	All	none	0	0-25	Low	Phosphorus
Fruit Juice	—	High Fructose Corn Syrup/Sucrose	11-5	0-15	61-510	Phosphorus, Vitamins C & A, B-vitamins, Calcium, Iron
Water	—	—	0	Low	Low	Low

Sources: Used by permission of the Gatorade Company.

contractions. Since sweating causes electrolyte losses (particularly sodium) as well as water losses, is it necessary to include electrolytes in fluid replacement beverages?

The argument against electrolyte replacement during exercise is that electrolyte needs can be more than adequately met by consuming a balanced diet. Also, since water loss during sweating is proportionately greater than electrolyte loss, the body's cells actually end up with a greater electrolyte concentration.

Although sodium is the principal mineral lost in sweat, our diets provide an abundance of salt — enough for any but extremely taxing exercise. The loss of 1 gram of sodium, which occurs with a 2-pound water loss, can be easily replaced by moderate salting of your food (½ teaspoon of salt provides 1 gram of sodium). Salt tablets should be avoided entirely — they can cause nausea due to irritation of the stomach lining, and can significantly increase your body's water requirement.

Potassium should not be a problem either — you lose far more sodium than potassium when you exercise. Orange juice, bananas, and potatoes are all excellent sources of potassium. Potassium supplements are un-necessary and can be dangerous. They can cause an excessively high level of potassium in the blood, resulting in an abnormal heart rhythm.

However, electrolyte deficits (particularly sodium) can occur under certain conditions — when you're acclimating to a hot environment, when you repeatedly work out in hot weather, or during ultra-endurance events like 50-mile runs, 100-mile bicycle rides and long triathlons, such as the Ironman.

Recent research* indicates that consuming only water during ultra-endurance events may produce a serious condition called *hyponatremia* (low blood sodium). Sodium losses in sweat during ultra-endurance events can be considerable, and drinking only water dilutes the amount

*JAMA, 772-774, 1986

of sodium left in the blood. Hyponatremic symptoms include lethargy, drowsiness, muscle twitching or cramping, muscle weakness, mental confusion and seizures. Fortunately, the condition is rare and can be easily prevented by consuming sports drinks containing sodium.

There is a concern that sports drinks contain too much sodium. Actually, there is a far smaller percentage of sodium in most sports drinks than in human sweat and a healthy person is at virtually no risk of incurring an electrolyte overload. In addition to aiding fluid absorption, the small amount of sodium in sports drinks encourages fluid intake because it makes the drink taste better. They also can restore fluid losses better than water because they replace plasma volume losses faster — important for both temperature regulation and performance.

Performance

If you're exercising hard for over an hour, then sports drinks can give you a performance edge that water can't. If you're exercising for less than this, however, water remains an effective and inexpensive fluid replacement beverage. As to which sports drink is best, basically it's a matter of choosing a beverage providing 6 to 8% carbohydrate, sodium, and avoiding drinks high in fructose. Otherwise, it's essentially a matter of personal preference.

Alcohol

Alcohol is occasionally promoted as an endurance aid. Proponents claim that alcohol consumption during exercise improves psychological well-being and/or aids proper hydration.

In fact, drinking alcohol prior to or during exercise can harm performance. Alcohol is a central nervous system

Figure 14
Adverse Effects of Dehydration

% Body Weight Loss	Symptoms
.5	Thirst
2.0	Stronger thirst, vague discomfort, loss of appetite
3.0	Increasing hemoconcentration, dry mouth, reduction in urine
4.0	Increased effort for exercise, flushed skin, impatience, apathy
5.0	Difficulty in concentrating
6.0	Impairment in exercise temperature regulation, increased HR
8.0	Dizziness, labored breathing in exercise, mental confusion
10.0	Spastic muscles, inability to balance with eyes closed, general incapacity, delirium and wakefulness, swollen tongue
11.0	Circulatory insufficiency, marked hemoconcentration and decreased blood volume, failing renal function

Source: J.E. Greenleaf, W.J. Fink. Fluid Intake and Athletic Performance IN *Nutrition and Athletic Performance* (W. Haskell, ed.). Bull Publishing Company, Palo Alto, CA, 1982. Used with permission.

depressant which reduces gross motor skills such as balance and coordination. It may decrease the output of glucose by the liver, leading to low blood glucose levels after prolonged endurance exercise. Alcohol consumption may also contribute to hypothermia (dangerously low body temperature) during prolonged exercise in cold weather. Also, alcohol, like caffeine, is a diuretic, which causes increased urination and water loss, which in turn can contribute to dehydration, particularly in hot weather.

Alcohol is a concentrated source of calories but does not contribute to the formation of muscle glycogen. One

12-ounce beer or 4-ounce glass of wine supplies only 50 calories of carbohydrate, enough to run a half mile. At the same time, these drinks supply .5 ounce of pure alcohol, a lot of potentially detrimental chemical with little effective fluid replacement. Finally, alcoholic beverages are high in calories and low in nutrients, and thus an "empty" source of calories for those who wish to reduce their body fat.

Twelve ounces of beer, 4 ounces of wine and 1½ ounces of distilled spirits contain about equal quantities of alcohol. One or two standard size drinks daily appear to cause no harm to healthy, non-pregnant adults if they can afford the calories. However, consumption of alcoholic beverages by pregnant women may cause birth defects or other problems during pregnancy. Since the level of consumption at which risks to the newborn occur has not been established, pregnant women should refrain from drinking. If you drink, substitute alcohol calories for fat and/or sugar calories, not food calories. One 12-ounce beer supplies 150 calories. A 4-ounce glass of wine or 1½ ounces of distilled spirits each provides 100 calories.

Chapter 10

The Sugar Debate
Poison or Pleasure?

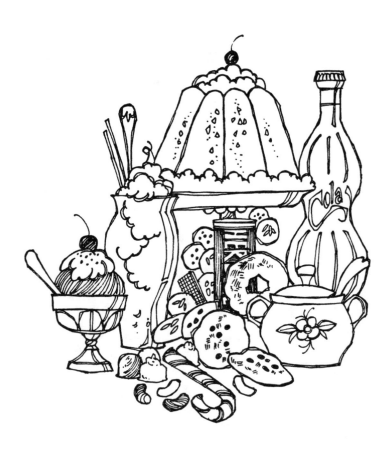

I was trying to finish the 200-mile ride in less than eleven hours. At the 130-mile mark, though, I weakened. I knew I needed food and accepted some glucose tablets from another rider. I probably ate 300 calories of straight glucose all at once.

Zap! Fifteen miles later I experienced severe gut cramps. For the last 50 miles the gas pains became so terrible I thought I would have to stop.

I must have had an awful fluid imbalance in my intestines. Though I achieved my goal, I would have felt much better if I had spaced those tablets out.

Sugar is not a poison. When eaten appropriately, it can be very helpful to the athlete. There are simple rules for how much to eat, when to eat it, and in what form.

Some athletes eat large quantities of sugar (and/or honey) in the belief that it is a high energy food and will improve endurance or speed. Others try to avoid it entirely, believing that sugar is detrimental to athletic performance and health. The better position is somewhere between these extremes.

Sugar Before Exercise

Athletes have been warned not to eat large amounts of sugar prior to exercise. This advice was based on the result of previous research* which indicated that consuming 75 grams of glucose (300 calories) 30 minutes prior to exercise reduced endurance by causing hypoglycemia (low blood sugar).

The explanation was that the sugar caused the pancreas to produce large amounts of insulin. Insulin lowers the blood sugar level, which is further lowered when the muscles pull glucose from the blood at the start of exercise. This combined lowering of the blood sugar was thought to explain the feelings of weakness, fatigue, and reduced endurance after the sugar feeding.

Newer research, however, contradicts the earlier findings**. Cyclists who consumed 300 calories of sugar

*Med Sci Sports, 11: 1-5, 1979
**Med Sci Sports Exerc, 19: 33-36, 1987

45 minutes prior to bicycling to exhaustion did as well as they did without the sugar feeding. There was no difference in performance even though the sugar feeding did raise their insulin level and lower their blood sugar.

Does this mean that it's okay to load up on soft drinks and candy (or more nutritional sources of sugar such as fruit juices and fruit) before exercise? Not necessarily. The results of both the old and new studies suggest that people differ in sensitivity to having their blood sugar lowered. While some people may feel weak and tired when their blood sugar drops during exercise, others will feel fine. The physiological basis for this difference is unknown.

On the basis of current knowledge, you should be advised that consuming sugar 30-45 minutes prior to exercise may harm your performance if you're sensitive to having your blood sugar lowered. You can test yourself subjectively in training to see if you develop any hypoglycemic symptoms (weakness, dizziness, nausea, confusion and partial black-out). Unless you have your blood sugar level directly measured, there is no objective way to determine if you have hypoglycemia.

Will consuming sugar before exercise help your performance? Recent research indicates it may if you're exercising longer than 90 minutes. In a study of cyclists*, those who consumed 220 calories of sugar (in solid or liquid form) five minutes before exercise performed better than those who did not have the sugar feeding.

Remember that you have enough muscle glycogen for at least 90 minutes of high intensity exercise. If you're exercising 90 minutes or longer, eating sugar prior to exercise provides glucose for your muscles to use when they're running low on glycogen. More on this when we discuss the pre-event meal in Chapter 12.

On the other hand, consuming sugar before anaerobic exercise such as sprinting or weight lifting will not improve

J Appl Physiol, 62:983-988, 1987

performance, because there is already enough ATP and muscle glycogen stored for these tasks. Nor will it help you to eat sugar before aerobic exercise lasting less than 90 minutes. It won't provide you with a sudden burst of energy, allowing you to exercise harder.

If you're concerned that you are sensitive to sugar feedings, consume the sugar either a few minutes prior to exercise, or wait until you're exercising. The rise in the exercise hormones (epinephrine and growth hormone) block the release of insulin, and counter insulin's effect in lowering blood sugar.

Sugar During Exercise

Carbohydrate feedings during endurance exercise lasting longer than 90 minutes may enhance endurance by providing glucose for muscles to use when their glycogen stores have dropped to low levels.

Utilizing its glycogen stores, the liver generally supplies glucose to maintain blood sugar for proper functioning of the central nervous system. As the muscles run out of glycogen during exercise, they will begin to take up some of the blood glucose, placing a drain on the liver glycogen stores. The longer the exercise session, the greater the utilization of blood glucose by the muscles for energy.

Though supplies of blood glucose are thus drawn from liver glycogen, muscle glycogen stays in the muscle and cannot provide glucose for the blood. When the liver glycogen is depleted, the blood glucose level drops. While some athletes experience hypoglycemic symptoms, most athletes are forced to reduce their exercise intensity due to muscular fatigue.

The improved performance associated with carbohydrate feedings during exercise is due to the maintenance of blood glucose levels. Dietary carbohydrate supplies glucose for the muscles at a time when their glycogen stores are diminished. Thus, carbohydrate use (and therefore ATP production) can continue at a high rate and endurance is enhanced. Remember that ATP (energy) production is faster from carbohydrate than from fat.

One study* measured performance during prolonged strenuous bicycling with and without carbohydrate feedings. During the ride without carbohydrate feeding, fatigue occurred after three hours and was preceded by a drop in blood glucose. During the ride when cyclists were fed carbohydrate, blood glucose levels were maintained and the cyclists were able to ride an additional hour before becoming fatigued.

How much carbohydrate should you consume during exercise to improve endurance? The research suggests taking in 25-30 grams (100-120 calories) every half hour. This amount can be obtained from carbohydrate-rich foods or from fluids.

Sports drinks are a practical source of carbohydrate, since they replace fluid losses as well. Eight ounces of a 6 to 8% carbohydrate sports drink every 15 minutes provides the proper amount of carbohydrate and helps maintain hydration.

Sugar During Training

Sugar can also be helpful for maintaining a high carbohydrate and calorie intake during training. If you train at a moderate level, say for an hour or so per day, carbohydrate should supply about 60% of the total calories in your diet. If you are in heavy training for two hours or more per day, carbohydrate should supply about 70% of your total calories. Complex carbohydrates should provide about half of your total calories. This means that during moderate training, sugar can provide 10% of your calories, and during heavy training, it can provide up to 20% of your total calories.

J Appl Physiol, 61:165-172, 1986

Keep in mind though, that sugar is a concentrated energy source but offers no other nutritional value. When sugar replaces complex carbohydrates in the diet, the intake of vitamins, minerals and fiber will be reduced. That is not a problem for a training athlete on a generous diet, provided it is sufficiently balanced to provide adequate nutrients and still carry the "empty calories" of sugar. (Also, remember that sugar can contribute to tooth decay.)

Forms of Sugar

Brown sugar, date sugar, honey and molasses are not nutritionally superior to table sugar. Though they do contain trace amounts of some vitamins and minerals, consumption of these so called "natural sugars" will not add significant nutritional value to your diet.

Some athletes take fructose thinking that it is superior to glucose or other sugars. Fructose causes a lower insulin response than glucose, which has lead some athletes to think that it is a superior energy source to glucose. However, consuming fructose does not improve endurance and has even been shown to harm performance. You store more muscle glycogen after eating starch or sucrose than when you eat fructose. Also, fructose is far more likely to cause gastrointestinal distress than glucose, even in small amounts. For this reason, glucose, sucrose and glucose polymers are the major carbohydrate sources in sports drinks.

Complex Carbohydrates

Your primary food source should be complex carbohydrates. They are important for athletic training and performance, and for health. They are good sources of vitamins, minerals and fiber.

The dietary fiber found in complex carbohydrates may reduce your risk for developing heart disease and cancer. Soluble fiber (fruits, vegetables, beans, oats and oat bran, and nuts) can help the cholesterol level in your blood. Since high blood cholesterol is one of the three major risk factors for heart disease, consuming more soluble fiber may help to reduce your risk for heart disease.

Insoluble fiber (whole grain bread/cereal products and bran) doesn't affect cholesterol, but may reduce your risk for bowel cancer and other intestinal diseases. Fruits and vegetables high in vitamins A and C may also help to prevent some kinds of cancer. Fiber also aids in satiety, important for weight control, and can help reduce constipation.

Compare a small baked potato with a third of a candy bar, which both contain about 100 calories. The potato provides ample vitamin C, with a small amount of protein, B vitamins, about half a dozen minerals, and fiber. The third of the candy bar provides the same amount of energy, almost three times as much fat, and little or no fiber, vitamins, or minerals.

Contrary to popular belief, starches such as bread, cereals, potatoes, corn, beans, rice and pasta contribute considerably less calories for a given amount than foods with a high fat or sugar content. (The "diet lunch" of a hamburger patty and a scoop of cottage cheese provides a lot of fat calories.)

By replacing fats and refined sugars in the diet, complex carbohydrates actually aid in weight control. Also, the naturally occurring sugars in fruit make them ideal for a sweet, low-calorie treat.

Eating too much sugar immediately before or during exercise will almost certainly cause gastrointestinal distress in the form of cramps, nausea, diarrhea and bloating.

Chapter 11

Caffeine

Unraveling the
Caffeine Controversy

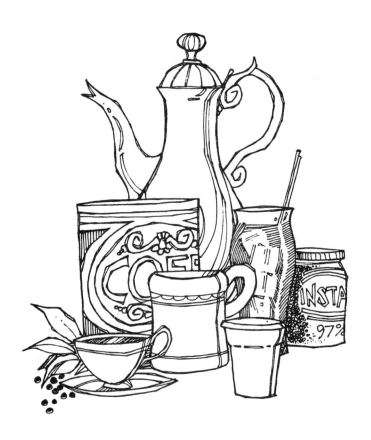

When the initial findings of the effects of caffeine were published, the man who presented the research was touted as a caffeine-pusher.

Those people who didn't drink coffee took issue with his findings.

Those people who had drunk coffee for years were elated that something good had been found in what they considered to be a bad habit.

Actually, he was an honest researcher who simply wanted to publish his findings without bias.

The use of caffeine to improve endurance is no longer an unsubstantiated theory. It can help some people, in certain circumstances. But it doesn't work for everyone — and there is a moral question for some.

Caffeine and the Availability of Fat

Since the depletion of muscle glycogen impairs endurance, the ability to burn fat as fuel instead of muscle glycogen will enhance endurance. As a rule, not enough fat is available in its usable form — free fatty acids — until late in exercise when your glycogen stores are already substantially reduced. So the goal is to increase the availability of fatty acids early in exercise.

When your muscles are presented with high levels of usable fat at the beginning of exercise, they will use more fat and less glycogen. One way to accomplish this is through endurance training itself, as I've discussed in Chapter 6. There is another possibility — consuming caffeine prior to exercise may also increase the availability of fat.

In one study*, 330 milligrams of caffeine (about two cups of strong coffee) were administered an hour prior to exercise, and the participants were able to exercise 19% longer before reaching exhaustion. The enhanced performance was directly related to a greater utilization of fat.

Caffeine stimulates adipose (fat) tissue to release fatty acids. Without the use of caffeine the study participants

Med Sc Sports, 10:155-158, 1978

obtained 22% of their energy from fat. After consuming caffeine, fat contributed almost 40% of the energy during exercise. This increased utilization of fat reduced the use of muscle glycogen and thus increased endurance. The participants also said the work seemed easier after the caffeine.

Effect on Exercise

It is not clear why the exercise seemed easier. There is no evidence that the perception of effort decreases because of increased fat utilization. But remember that caffeine is a stimulant, and that may explain the lower perceived exertion rating. As a stimulant, caffeine may lower the threshold for muscle fiber recruitment and neural transmission, making it easier to recruit muscle fibers for work.

In another study*, consuming a caffeinated drink before and during two hours of exercise increased the work production by 7.4%, providing evidence that intensity as well as endurance is enhanced by caffeine.

The results of these studies suggest that you might be able to exercise longer and/or complete a given workload in a shorter time period. They also suggest that you need to exercise *longer than an hour* to benefit from caffeine.

Caffeine exerts its influence by indirectly causing the adipose tissue to break down fat so that fatty acids are released into the bloodstream. It does this by interfering with a substance that stops the breakdown of fat. (Several of the body's hormones influence the adipose tissue in a similar way to cause the breakdown of fat.)

Med Sci Sports, 11:6-11, 1979

Figure 15
Sources of Caffeine

Coffee (5-oz. cup)

Espresso	150 mg.
Drip	110-150 mg.
Percolator	64-124 mg.
Instant	40-108 mg.
Decaffeinated (instant)	2 mg.
Decaffeinated (brewed)	2-5 mg.

Chocolate

6 oz. cocoa	10 mg.
1 oz. milk chocolate	6 mg.
1 oz. baking chocolate	35 mg.
1 oz. bittersweet chocolate	20 mg.
8 oz. chocolate milk	10 mg.

Soft Drinks (12 ounces)

Diet Mr. Pibb	59 mg.
Mountain Dew	54 mg.
Mellow Yellow	53 mg.
Tab	47 mg.
Coca-Cola, Diet Coke	46 mg.
Shasta Cola, Diet Cola	44 mg.
Shasta Cherry Cola	44 mg.
Shasta Diet Cherry Cola	44 mg.
Sunkist Orange	42 mg.
Mr Pibb	41 mg.
Dr. Pepper	40 mg.
Sugar-free Dr. Pepper	40 mg.
Big Red	38 mg.
Pepsi	38 mg.
Diet Pepsi, Pepsi Light	36 mg.
Royal Crown Cola	36 mg.
Diet Rite	36 mg.
Canada Dry Jamaica Cola	30 mg.
Canada Dry Diet Cola	1 mg.
Cragmont Cola	Trace
7-Up, Diet 7-Up	0 mg.
Sprite, Fresca	0 mg.
RC-100	0 mg.
Diet Sunkist	0 mg.
Fanta Orange	0 mg.
Hires Root Beer	0 mg.

Tea (5-oz. cup)

Black tea brewed 5 min.	20-50 mg.
Black tea brewed 3 min.	20-46 mg.
Black tea brewed 1 min.	9-33 mg.
Green tea	30 mg.
Instant tea	12-28 mg.
Ice tea (12 oz. can)	22-36 mg.

Drugs (per tablet)

Pain Relivers

Excedrin	64-130 mg.
Anacin, Emprin, or Vanquish	32 mg.
Aspirin (plain)	0 mg.

Feminine Needs

Pre Mens Forte	100 mg.
Pre Mens	66 mg.
Midol	32-65 mg.
Cope	32 mg.

Allergy/Cold Remedies

Dristan	16 mg.
Triaminicin	30 mg.
Coryban-D	30 mg.

Diuretic

Aqua-Ban	200 mg.
Permathene	200 mg.

Diet/Weight Control:

Dexatrim	200 mg.
Dietac	200 mg.
Prolamine	140 mg.

Alertness/Stimulants

Vivarin	200 mg.
No Doz	100-200 mg.

Prescription

Cafergot	100 mg.
Migralam	100 mg.
Firorinal	40 mg.
Esgic	40 mg.
Aspectol	32 mg.
Darvon	32 mg.

Source: *Maximize Your Body Potential,* by Joyce D. Nash, Ph.D., Bull Publishing Company, Palo Alto, CA. Used with permission. Products change from time to time, and caffeine content may also change.

When and How Much

The best results are achieved by consuming 4 to 5 milligrams of caffeine per kilogram of body weight one hour prior to exercise. This is equivalent to about two 6-ounce cups of coffee for a 154-pound person.

If you decide to try caffeine, experiment with it in training first. Some people are extremely sensitive to caffeine and won't perform better with it. Also, exceeding the 5-milligram dose won't provide additional benefits and may cause caffeine toxicity — nausea, muscle tremor and headache. Sensitive people may experience these side effects at lower doses. Elite athletes will probably not benefit as much from caffeine, because they already have an increased ability to mobilize fat during exercise.

Keep in mind that caffeine is a diuretic. In hot weather, excessive caffeine can stimulate the production of urine and cause water losses. This may contribute to dehydration and reduced endurance.

Another word of caution — not all research studies have shown that caffeine improves endurance. It may not for you. Those studies showing that caffeine improves performance and reduces muscle glycogen utilization have used cyclists as subjects. Whether or not caffeine improves performance for other endurance sports is questionable.

The Moral Issue

There is also a moral question. The use of caffeine tablets or coffee can be considered a form of doping. On the one hand, people have been drinking coffee for years as a regular part of their diets. On the other hand, the amount of caffeine that is needed to exert the best effect (4 to 5 milligrams per kilogram) represents a pharmacological dose. The American College of Sports Medicine, the United States Olympic Committee, and the American Dietetic Association don't endorse the use of caffeine to enhance endurance.

The measure of doping established by the International Olympic Committee (IOC) is a urine caffeine concentration greater than 12 micrograms per milliliter. This standard is higher than concentrations expected from caffeine doses normally used to enhance performance. You would have to drink six to eight cups of coffee in one sitting and be tested within two to three hours to reach this standard.

The use of caffeine has become controversial. It requires individual evaluation and judgment.

Chapter 12

Eating for Performance
The High-Performance Diet

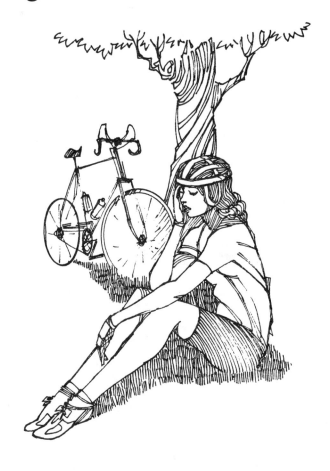

It was the last rest stop, the 170-mile mark of a 200-mile cycling race. We had been riding for ten hours — four of those hours in 90-degree heat.

I was sunburned, breathing hard, hurting. Lying on the ground I ate about five chocolate chip cookies, wondering if I could ride another 30 miles. My chief adversary rode up and my heart sank — she looked great.

We had been riding neck and neck and she seemed definitely to be the stronger one. I knew that she hadn't taken a rest or eaten since the 150-mile mark. "C'mon," she said to a friend. "Let's go in and pick up my trophy."

I dragged myself back onto my bike and gave chase. It was sheer determination and concentration on my part that kept my legs moving. My competitor was talking and making jokes, looking like she was part of her cycle.

About ten miles later she began to fade as I perked up. "What's the matter?" I asked her.

"I don't know," she said. "I feel weak and shaky."

Slowly the roles reversed. I felt strong. She faded off the back of the pace line. I pulled the pace line into the finish for the last 15 miles — finishing strongly and feeling great.

Later, I learned that my competitor had stopped about ten miles out. She ordered a shake at a fast food restaurant and fainted. It had been two and one-half to three hours since she had eaten.

There is a great deal of confusion about what, if anything, to eat before and during competition. To some degree it is an individual matter. Only you can truly learn what works for you — by trial and error well before competition. The length of your event also makes a difference; there are guidelines for events of varying duration.

Pre-Exercise Eating

During exercise, you rely primarily on your pre-existing muscle glycogen and fat stores. Although the pre-exercise meal doesn't contribute immediate energy for exercise, it can provide energy when you exercise for longer than an hour and a half.

Athletes often train or compete in the morning without eating. This overnight fast lowers your liver glycogen stores (the body's main source of blood glucose) and can impair performance, especially if you attempt to train or compete in a prolonged endurance event (over 90 minutes) that relies heavily on blood glucose.

Athletes are often discouraged from eating prior to exercise. The rationale is that if any food remains in the stomach when you start exercising, you can become nauseated when blood is diverted from the stomach to the exercising muscles.

Before competition, most athletes are tense, which slows the transit time of food. A distended stomach may also restrict breathing. Thus, athletes are usually advised to eat two to three hours prior to exercise, to allow adequate time for stomach emptying. Rather than get up at the crack of dawn to eat, those who train or compete in the morning often prefer to forgo eating.

Athletes have also been instructed to avoid high-carbohydrate foods immediately before exercising. The concern is that carbohydrate may elevate blood insulin at the start of exercise, resulting in hypoglycemia and fatigue during the exercise.

Actually, as discussed in Chapter 10, eating carbohydrate before exercise probably won't harm performance unless the individual is sensitive to a lowering of blood glucose. Again, however, you should test the effectiveness of the pre-exercise meal in training, not before an important competition.

Eating a high-carbohydrate meal before morning exercise can help restore reduced liver glycogen stores, which will help performance during prolonged exercise (over 90 minutes). If muscle glycogen stores are low, the meal can help to increase them as well if you eat several hours before exercise.

How much carbohydrate should you consume in the pre-exercise meal? The research* suggests 1 to 4 grams of carbohydrate per kilogram of body weight, consumed one to four hours before exercise.

Admittedly, this provides a wide range of amounts and time, and the key is to relate the amount you eat to the time lapse. To avoid potential gastrointestinal distress, the size of the meal should be reduced the closer to exercise it is consumed. For example, a carbohydrate feeding of 1 gram per kilogram (4 calories per kilogram) is appropriate an hour before exercise, whereas 4 grams per kilogram (16 calories per kilogram) can be consumed four hours before exercise.

Good examples of solid high-carbohydrate foods for pre-exercise meals include fruit, bread products (adding

Med Sci Sports Exerc, 21: 598-604, 1989

jam or jelly increases the carbohydrate content) and non-fat or low-fat yogurt. Fruit juices and non-fat milk are good high-carbohydrate beverages. You can also use high-carbohydrate liquid supplements.

Fat should be limited because it slows food transit time and for many people gives a feeling of heaviness or sluggishness. In contrast, carbohydrates provide the quickest and most efficient source of energy and, unlike fats, are rapidly digested. Remember that many high-protein foods (eggs, cheese) are also high in fat.

Liquid Meals

A number of commercially formulated liquid meals are also available (see Figure 16). They are high in carbohydrate and also provide fluid. They have several advantages over conventional meals.

Liquid meals leave the stomach more rapidly than regular meals and thus may help to avoid pre-competition nausea.

They also produce a low stool residue, and thus help keep immediate weight gain to a minimum. Because of their low residue, liquid meals are also less likely to necessitate a bathroom break during exercise. (While this is merely annoying during training, it can be disastrous during competition).

Liquid meals can also be used for nutritional supplementation during heavy training when caloric requirements are very high. They contribute a significant number of calories as well as a feeling of satiety. They may also be used as an energy source during prolonged exercise.

Home-made liquid meals can be concocted by mixing milk, fruit, and non-fat dry milk powder in a blender. For added variety, cereal, yogurt, and flavoring (vanilla and chocolate) can be added. Sugar or honey may also be added for additional sweetness and carbohydrate.

Figure 16
Nutritional Beverage Comparison Chart

Beverage	Flavors	Calories per 8 oz. serving	Carbohydrate (grams)	Fat (grams)	Protein (grams)
GatorPro™ The Quaker Oats Company	Chocolate, Strawberry, Vanilla	360	58 (65%)	7 (17%)	16 (18%)
Exceed® Ross Laboratories	Chocolate, Strawberry, Vanilla	360	54 (60%)	9.5 (24%)	14 (16%)
Nutrament® Mead Johnson Nutritionals	Chocolate, Banana, Vanilla, Strawberry, Coconut	240	34 (57%)	6.5 (25%)	11 (18%)
Go™ Nutri-Products, Inc.	Chocolate, Strawberry, Vanilla	190	27 (56%)	3 (13%)	15 (31%)
Sustacal® Mead Johnson Nutritionals	Chocolate, Vanilla, Strawberry, Egg Nog	240	33 (55%)	5.5 (21%)	14.5 (24%)
SportShake Mid-America Farms	Chocolate	310	45 (58%)	10 (29%)	11 (13%)
Sego® Pet, Inc.	Chocolate, Strawberry, Vanilla	180	27 (60%)	4 (20%)	9 (20%)

Source: Used by permission of the Gatorade Company.

Exercise Lasting 90 Minutes or Less

The recommended training diet for moderate training (48% carbohydrate, 10% sugar, 12% protein and 30% fat) provides adequate muscle glycogen stores for exercise of any intensity which lasts 90 minutes or less. Carbohydrate loading won't improve performance, and may harm it because of the feeling of stiffness and heaviness sometimes associated with increased muscle glycogen stores.

Eating immediately before exercise should be an individual choice — just follow the general pre-exercise meal guidelines to avoid problems. Caffeine ingestion may allow you to exercise harder, particularly if you're exercising for an hour or more. Proper hydration should be the major nutritional concern during exercise of any appreciable length. There have been cases of heat exhaustion and heat stroke in runs as short as 6.2 miles. Sports drinks may give you a boost if you're exercising longer than an hour.

Exercise Lasting 90 Minutes to Three Hours

You can carbohydrate load (as discussed in Chapter 5) to increase your muscle glycogen stores in the days prior to competition. (Keep in mind that training too heavily the week prior to competition can predispose you to early muscle glycogen depletion.) You can also consume caffeine (as discussed in Chapter 11) to slow down the rate of glycogen utilization during training and competition. Also, eating before exercise may contribute energy towards the end of the exercise.

When you're exercising two hours or more per day, you should consume the diet recommended for heavy training — approximately 70% carbohydrates (no more than 20% from sugar), 12% from protein, and the balance from fat. This will help prevent training glycogen depletion, as discussed in Chapter 4.

Figure 17
Food/Fluid for Events of Varying Length

Length of Event

Dietary Intake	0-90 minutes	1½-3 hours	3 hours and up
Pre-exercise meal 1-4 hours before exercise	Probably will not help	May improve endurance	May improve endurance
Caffeine	May help beyond 60 minutes	May improve endurance	May improve endurance
Sports drinks with 6-8% carbohydrate	May help beyond 60 minutes	May improve endurance	May improve endurance
Carbohydrate loading	May harm performance due to weight gain	May improve endurance	May improve endurance
High carbohydrate foods/ "liquid meals" during exercise	Probably will not help	May improve endurance— sports drinks better choice	May improve endurance— provides a variety

During exercise your primary need is fluid. Try various sports drinks if you want, and any addition to the fluid that suits you the best. Keep in mind that sports drinks can improve your endurance when you exercise longer than 60 minutes by providing carbohydrate for the exercising muscles.

When you're exercising over 90 minutes, you should consume 25 to 30 grams of carbohydrate every half hour to improve endurance (as discussed in Chapter 10). This amount can be obtained through carbohydrate-rich foods or sports drinks. High-carbohydrate foods include fruit, grain products (e.g., graham crackers, bagels), liquid meals, and sports bars. Start taking in carbohydrate early, within the first half-hour of exercise.

Three Hours and Beyond

Again, you can carbohydrate load before competition and ingest caffeine before both training and competition to improve endurance. During training, you should eat the recommended diet for heavy training.

When you exercise for three hours or longer, the food and fluid you consume before and during the exercise is at least as important as what you have eaten the week before. When you're exercising this long, you need carbohydrate to provide glucose for the working muscles. It will also prevent susceptible athletes from developing hypoglycemic symptoms.

As outlined earlier, you can get carbohydrate from sports drinks, and from high-carbohydrate foods — fruit, grain products, sports bars, and liquid meals. These foods should be easily digestible, familiar (what you are used to eating in training) and enjoyable (to encourage you to eat).

Stay away from foods high in fat and protein, because they are harder to digest. Any food that is hard to digest will cause competition between your stomach and muscles for blood, and possible nausea and vomiting.

Eat before you feel tired or hungry, within 30 minutes into exercise. If you eat small amounts at frequent intervals (every 30 to 60 minutes), you'll be more likely to prevent gastrointestinal upsets.

Once again, proper hydration is the most important nutritional concern during prolonged exercise. You can have adequate muscle glycogen stores and blood glucose and still collapse from heat exhaustion or stroke. Consume fluids before you are thirsty, as early as 15 minutes into exercise, and continue drinking according to a set schedule, as discussed in Chapter 9.

Never try an untested food or fluid during competition. The result may be severe indigestion and/or impaired performance.

After Exercise

Weigh yourself after exercising and drink 16 ounces of fluid for each pound lost. Remember that you also require carbohydrate to replace the glycogen you used during exercise. You will recover faster if you eat a high-carbohydrate diet (60-70% calories from carbohydrate).

The time period in which carbohydrate is consumed relative to exercise is also important. One study* compared glycogen replacement when carbohydrate was consumed immediately after exercise to replacement when carbohydrate consumption was delayed for two hours after exercise. When carbohydrate feeding was delayed for two hours, glycogen storage was cut in half (when measured four hours after exercise).

J Appl Physiol, 65:1480-1485, 1988

This means that delaying carbohydrate intake for too long after exercise will reduce muscle glycogen storage and impair recovery. Many people aren't hungry after exercising. If this is the case, consume a high-carbohydrate drink such as fruit juice or a commercial high-carbohydrate beverage. This will also help rehydration.

How much carbohydrate should you take in after exercise? The research suggests consuming 1 to 1.5 grams of carbohydrate per kilogram of body weight (4 to 6 calories per kilogram) within 30 minutes of exercise, followed by similar amounts every two to four hours thereafter. The first carbohydrate feeding could be a high-carbohydrate beverage and the following feedings could be high-carbohydrate meals.

For example, following exercise, a 70-kilogram man should take in 70 to 105 grams of carbohydrate within 30 minutes. This amount corresponds to 12 to 18 ounces of GatorLode®. Two hours later, he has 2 cups of spaghetti with ½ cup of tomato sauce, which provides 70 grams of carbohydrate. Adding two pieces of French bread increases his carbohydrate intake to 100 grams.

Chapter 13

Body Composition
Debunking the Myth
of Bathroom Scales

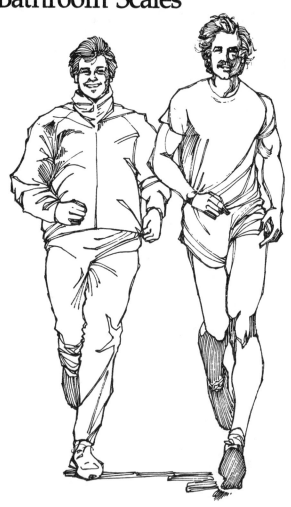

I worked with a muscular, well-built man about 5'7", 150 pounds, who decided that if he were thinner he could run better. He had looked at a height-weight table and decided that he should weigh 135 pounds.

He cut his food intake, but kept his mileage the same. Not only did he have a difficult time losing weight, but his running form deteriorated. He lost his power and speed. He also became irritable, hungry and began to fantasize about banana cream pie.

I evaluated his body composition and learned that at 150 pounds he had 7% body fat. I told him to throw his bathroom scale out the window and go back to his old diet. Soon, his running form returned to normal.

We are a society obsessed about our weight. How many people do you know who would not give high priority to "just losing a few pounds"? It carries over to athletics — with target weights for everyone.

What really counts is body composition: the relative amounts of lean body mass and fat. We should pay attention to percent body fat, if we want to maximize our potential. We may even find we should gain a few pounds.

The True Measure of Fatness

In our society, the bathroom scale has a following worthy of a political party or religion. An unbelievable number of weight loss gimmicks have been spawned by the American obsession about losing weight. Some of them endanger the health of their victims, others merely thin wallets, and almost all fail to cause permanent weight loss. In the rush to shed pounds, a very important question is usually overlooked: "How fat am I?"

The scale cannot differentiate between fat pounds and muscle pounds. People automatically assume that a gain in scale weight represents fat weight and that a loss in scale weight is fat loss. Thus, you often hear someone exclaim, "I've lost six pounds in one day!" It's physiologically impossible to lose six pounds of fat in one day. That someone has actually lost water — which will be replaced. Fluctuations in scale weight do not necessarily represent changes in body fat, and that's what counts.

The scale does not indicate how fat a person is because both fat and muscle (and some other things, including water) contribute to the total weight. The term "over-weight" only refers to body weight in excess of the average weight for a specific height. The term "underweight" only refers to the body weight below the average weight for height.

The scale is prejudiced against stocky, muscular people just as it is biased in favor of thin, slightly built people. What tells the tale is not total weight but body composition.

Body composition divides weight into two categories. One is lean body mass, of which muscle is the major component. The other category is fat. What is really important is how much of a person's weight is fat. This is expressed as *percent body fat*.

Types of Body Builds

Appearances can be very deceptive when it comes to estimating percent body fat. When comparing the total fat of a marathon runner to that of a football player, most people would say that the marathon runner has less fat because he looks thinner. Yet, when evaluated, the football player may be as lean, in terms of percent body fat, as the runner.

Sure, the football player appears to be fatter, but this is because he is bigger. His weight and size are due to his enormous muscle mass. The runner, who in comparison may look like a prisoner of war, has proportionately less muscle mass. It is possible for two people to be 100 pounds apart in weight and have totally different body types, yet have the same percent body fat.

As I said above, the person who suffers the most when evaluated by weight alone is the stocky, muscular type. Though this person may have little fat, he or she weighs more than the average because of a large lean body mass. The body fat may be so low that to lose weight the person would almost have to lose muscle. When such a person loses weight by dieting, much of the loss may actually be of muscle, with a resulting deterioration in performance.

Body shape and size are largely determined by skeleton size; a certain amount of muscle and tissue accompany a certain amount of bone. The total amount and the distribution of muscle mass will depend to some degree on the athlete's chosen sport (and type of training). For example, weight training will increase muscle mass more than long distance running.

As athletes know, body type is important in most sports, and each sport seems to require a distinctive body type. The large, muscular person will never be an elite marathoner, just as the elite marathoner would not survive as an interior lineman on the football field. Each athlete has a genetic profile that largely determines his limits for both body build and composition.

Body Composition

You are thus somewhat restricted by your genetic inheritance, but this does not mean that you can't improve yourself. While body build and size may be altered only slightly, substantial change may occur in body composition. Such changes can have a significant effect on your performance.

In some sports, performance may be negatively affected by excess muscle gained from weight lifting. It is also obvious that endurance performance is impaired by excess body fat. However, the athlete who trains for a specific sport by doing it, or at least simulating the physical activity involved will have the muscle mass that is, for him, suited to that sport. If because of his genetic inheritance, his muscle mass is greater than he desires, he will only hurt himself by trying to starve himself thinner.

The target percent body fat for men for general health is 15%. A man is classified as fat when he has 20% body fat and obese when he exceeds 24% body fat. The desirable level of body fat for women for general health is 22%. A woman is classified as fat when she has 27% body fat and obese when she exceeds 31% body fat.

People who regularly participate in endurance exercise such as running, bicycling and swimming usually have lower percentages of body fat, because the exercise both increases their lean body mass and uses up stored fat as fuel. Some authorities suggest that a male endurance athlete in top condition should not exceed 8% body fat.

Three percent of the total body fat in men is considered "essential fat." It appears that a man cannot reduce his body fat below this limit without impairing his physiological function and capacity for exercise. The body fat of world class male marathoners ranges from about 4 to 8%, which is only slightly above the level of fat essential for health.

In contrast to men, the amount of body fat a top female endurance athlete should carry is less clear. The percent body fat considered "essential" for women is 12%. This higher level of fat is related to child bearing functions and takes into account sex specific fat in the breasts and other tissues. One study of elite female distance runners found that all were below 18% body fat. Some were even below the essential body fat limit of 12%*.

Generally, women should not reduce their total percent body fat below 10 to 12%, probably the lower desirable limit for women in good health. But if a woman is serious about competing in endurance sports, she should probably not exceed 15% body fat. Extra fat weight, unlike extra muscle weight, just adds to the mass to be moved and does not assist in propelling the body.

*Med Sci Sports, 6:178-181, 1974

Obviously, no matter how low your percent body fat, your success in an endurance sport will depend on a variety of factors. Having a low percent body fat does not, in itself, insure you will be an elite athlete.

Before you attempt to achieve a certain percent body fat, there are several things to bear in mind. The recommendations for athletes in top condition (8% for men and 15% or less for women) do not hold true for every person. One can generalize that you should definitely be at or below the generally desirable levels of 15% for men and 22% for women, but beyond that, your ideal percent body fat is where you perform the best. Attempting to reach an unrealistic percent body fat can set you back just as much as shooting for an unrealistic weight.

Assessing Body Composition

People who start an exercise program should have periodic body fat assessments. If you lose two pounds of fat but gain two pounds of muscle, your weight will not change, even though you'll be thinner. This occurs frequently when a previously inactive person begins to exercise. Because muscle is denser than fat, and thus takes up less room, you'll appear to have lost weight; in fact you'll be thinner.

It is even possible to gain weight while losing fat because of correspondingly greater muscle gain. For example, you could lose two pounds of fat but gain four pounds of muscle. This often happens to sedentary women who begin an exercise program. They may drop two dress sizes but gain two pounds. Some have even quit exercising when this happens because they're conditioned to go by scale weight. Talk about worshiping false gods! Rather than becoming unnerved by scale fluctuations, get your body evaluated.

Body composition can be determined in many ways, but two of the most accurate and practical are by underwater

Figure 18
Body Composition Values of Male and Female Athletes

Sport	Male	Female
Baseball	12-15%	na
Basketball	7-11%	21%
Bicycling	9%	15%
Gymnastics	5%	10-17%
Football	14%	na
Swimming	5-11%	17-24%
Running (distance)	5-8%	15-18%
Triathlon	7%	13%
Body Builders	8%	13%
Wrestling	5-10%	na
Volleyball	12%	18%
Tennis	15%	20%

Source: Adapted from J.H. Willmore and D. L. Costill, *Training for Sport and Activity: The Physiological Basis of the Conditioning Process*, 3rd edition. Boston, Allyn and Bacon, 1988.

weighing and with measurements using skinfold calipers. Each method has advantages as well as inherent problems, and special training is required to assure accuracy. When administered by trained personnel, however, both tests give good indications of percent body fat. Some sports medicine facilities and colleges offer body composition evaluation (as well as $\dot{V}O_{2max}$ testing).

Bioelectrical impedance is a new and popular technique to determine body fat. Impedance involves passing a small electrical current throughout the body and measuring the resistance encountered. Lean tissue is a good conductor of electricity; fat is not. Unfortunately, impedance tends to overestimate the body fat of a lean person and under-estimate the body fat of an obese person.

Chapter 14

No Convenient Way to Lose Weight

Permanent Weight Control Can Only Be Achieved Through Lifelong Exercise

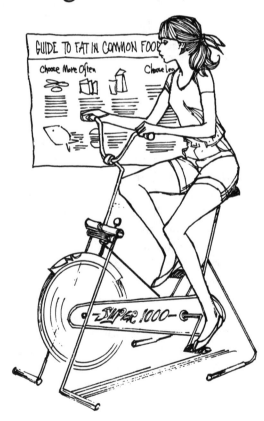

A professional person with a desk job wanted to lose weight. She tried every fad diet but could never keep the pounds off.

She tried a sensible diet — well-balanced with a calorie deficit — but it didn't work, either.

Finally, a fitness enthusiast got her walking for 30 minutes a day. She very slowly lost weight at a rate of about two pounds a month. She also found that she wasn't as hungry as before, and that she could even eat a larger quantity of food, while still controlling her weight.

Weight loss is equated to counting calories. The calories in our food are an important factor in weight control, but as every jaded dieter (most of the country) knows, it's more complicated than that.

We are just beginning to understand how important exercise is for any weight control program. The statistics are mounting, that show a consistent connection between successful weight control and regular exercise. And we are learning more about why this is so.

Weight Control and Energy Balance

The energy sources in food, as well as the body's energy expenditure, are measured in units of heat expressed as *kilocalories* — abbreviated *calories*. Protein and carbohydrate both supply 4 calories per gram, fat supplies 9 calories per gram (and alcohol 7 calories per gram).

Maintaining weight, gaining weight, or losing weight is all a matter of energy balance: Your body weight will stay the same when your caloric intake equals your caloric output; it will change when there is an imbalance between caloric expenditure and caloric intake.

To gain weight, energy intake must be greater than energy output. To lose weight, energy output must be greater than energy intake. In short, if you want to lose weight, you must eat less, exercise more, or both.

The Importance of Exercise

Although caloric restriction is usually chosen over exercise as a means of weight loss, exercise is more effective than dieting for reducing body fat. This is due to the fundamental fact that diet and exercise have different effects on metabolic rate. Diets that are too low in calories reduce metabolic rate (the idling rate of your body, which affects how many calories you use up apart from exercise). Since the dieter needs less calories, less weight is lost. This commonly leads to the "plateau phase," where weight loss slows or even ceases, even though the dieter is still counting calories. Often this leads to frustration — and the end of the diet. If the basic metabolic rate drops, caloric intake must be reduced by a like amount to maintain weight loss — a demanding situation for even the most dedicated dieter.

Exercise tends to increase the metabolic rate. This effect persists even after exercise. For example, the metabolic rate may remain elevated after moderate exercise (60% $\dot{V}O_{2max}$ or 70% maximum heart rate) lasting only 40 to 60 minutes. This added energy expenditure, often well after exercise, is not taken into account on the charts which list caloric expenditure from different activities. The added calories equal about 5 to 8% of the caloric cost of the activity*. Although small, this increased caloric expenditure — over and above the energy cost of the exercise itself — can aid weight loss over a period of time.

Dieting causes losses of both body fat and lean body tissue. With extreme caloric restrictions, involving semi-starvation or complete fasting, as much as a third of the weight lost may come from lean body mass. (Some of these severe effects have been reduced by the newest "protein sparing" regimens, utilizing well-balanced nutrient supplements.) Even a sensible, well-balanced diet, where no more than two pounds is lost per week, may cause some muscle loss. But the amount of muscle lost on such a program is minimal compared to that lost on drastic unsupervised diet regimens.

Med Sci Sports Exerc, 18: 205-210, 1986

Exercise and Appetite

Exercise is of course the critical factor, promoting both fat loss and increase in muscle mass. However, sedentary people often avoid exercise for weight loss, believing that it will increase their appetite and counteract the energy-using effects of the exercise. It doesn't work out that way.

When considering the effect of exercise on food intake, you must account for the intensity and duration of activity. Obviously, athletes who spend many hours in vigorous training each day will eat more than if they were sedentary, but they stay quite lean, in terms of body fat percentage. Actually, sedentary people eat slightly more than those who engage in light to moderate activity for up to an hour each day*. Exercise within this range appears to be a mild appetite suppressant.

Using Exercise Effectively

Another misconception is that it takes an excruciating amount of exercise to lose an appreciable amount of body fat. For example, people tend to focus on statements to the effect that you would have to run 35 miles to lose one pound of fat. The point lost is that that is not how people exercise — the goal is comfortable increments, however modest, and the calorie expending effects will add up. A 3,500 calorie deficit equals one pound of fat, whether this happens rapidly or gradually over a period of time. Patience pays — this kind of gradual weight loss (from fat) is more permanent than losses from extreme diets.

Caloric restriction by itself, then, has proved ineffective over the long run for many people. When dieting is combined with exercise, however, it accomplishes several things: fat loss can occur more rapidly than when either dieting or exercise is used alone; combining the two

*Amer J Clin Nutr, 4:169-175, 1956

reduces the proportion of weight lost from lean tissue; and exercise can reduce the tendency of dieting to lower the metabolic rate. It also furnishes another option for the jaded dieter who is sick of counting calories — with exercise added in, he can increase food intake, yet achieve fat loss, by exercising longer, harder or more days per week.

A Sensible Diet

The American College of Sports Medicine has provided guidelines for desirable weight loss programs. Adults should consume at least 1,200 calories to meet nutritional requirements.

The daily caloric deficit can range from 500 to 1,000 calories, depending on the person's caloric requirement. This mild caloric restriction results in a manageable potential loss of water, electrolytes, minerals, and lean body mass, and is unlikely to cause malnutrition.

The rate of sustained loss should not exceed two pounds per week (3,500 calories equals one pound of fat). An effective weight control program also incorporates aerobic exercise, the preferred type for maximum benefit.

Behavior modification techniques should also be used to identify and eliminate eating habits that contribute to excess calories. The lifestyle changes must be realistic, since successful weight control requires a lifelong commitment.

The low-fat, high-complex carbohydrate diet recommended by the U.S. Dietary Goals promotes fat loss for several reasons. Since fat is a concentrated source of calories, reducing fat intake will reduce caloric intake.

Fat is also more fattening than carbohydrate because dietary fat is more likely to be stored as body fat. The conversion of dietary carbohydrate to body fat is metabolically costly — about 23% of the carbohydrate calories are expended in the conversion process. The conversion of dietary fat to body fat is easy and requires little energy —

about 3% of the fat calories are expended in the conversion process*.

The Exercise Prescription

The exercise prescription for weight control is similar to that for improving cardio-respiratory (endurance) fitness. This involves participating in aerobic exercise (such as walking, jogging, bicycling, swimming or aerobic dance) three to five days per week at moderate intensity (50 to 80% of aerobic capacity, 60-90% of maximum heart rate), for 20 to 60 minutes continuously.

The goal should be to expend at least 300 calories per session, since this seems to represent a threshold for body fat loss. If the intensity of the exercise is low, you do it longer, until the 300 calories have been expended. In practical terms, 300 calories is roughly equal to a typical aerobics class session, walking or jogging three miles, bicycling 12 miles or swimming one mile. Because total energy expenditure is closely related to fat loss, increased frequency, intensity and/or duration of training should cause proportionately greater reductions in body fat.

Although fat can also be reduced through anaerobic exercise like sprinting or interval training, the exercise usually doesn't last long enough to achieve a caloric deficit comparable to that realized with aerobic exercise. Most people who use anaerobic workouts are trying to increase their speed rather than lose body fat. Those who are unfit and engage in anaerobic exercise usually find it unpleasant and stop exercising altogether. There have been too many cases of unfit people sprinting once around a quarter mile track (and leaving the joggers in their wake), only to nearly collapse and never return to exercise.

* *J Clin Invest*, 79: 1019-1025, 1987.

Eating Tips

If you feel that you're exercising enough but eating too much, you can decrease your caloric intake by eating fewer "empty calories" — foods high in sugar and fat, and alcohol. You can improve your eating habits through some simple techniques, such as preparing smaller portions, eating more slowly, and avoiding seconds.

The meal frequency of your diet is also important. Skipping meals earlier in the day is more likely to cause over-eating in the evening, so eating regular meals can aid in weight control.

Spot Reducing

If you hope to spot reduce, you're in for disappointment. Exercise, even when localized, draws from all the fat stores of the body, not just from the local fat depots. Your body has its own ideas about where it wants to store fat, and unfortunately these tend to be the "wrong" places. (One example would be tennis players who have been found to have the same triceps skinfold on both arms, even though their dominant arm was exercised more.)

Exercising a specific area does increase the muscle tone in that area. For example, substantial reductions in abdominal girth, up to three to four inches, can result from localized exercise like sit-ups. This is not due to fat loss. Rather, the abdominal muscles are strengthened and better able to pull your abdomen back to where you want it.

Spot reduction is often promoted to eliminate the so-called "cellulite" in specific areas of the body. Cellulite doesn't exist — it's just a gimmicky name for subcutaneous fat. Stay away from any sales pitch that uses the term.

Focus on Body Fat Percentage

Keep in mind that the desirable percent body fat for general health for men and women is 15% and 22%, respectively. If you are overweight (by height-weight table standards), due to a large lean body mass, but not overfat, relax. If you are overweight and overfat, either use exercise alone or combine a mild-to-moderate calorie restriction with an aerobic exercise program. This will insure that any weight loss is from fat. If you're overfat but not overweight, due to a small lean body mass, skip the diet and shape up with aerobic exercise.

Usually weight changes little, if any, in the first few weeks of an exercise program. This is because lean weight initially increases at about the same rate that fat weight is being lost. You can become discouraged, because the scales show no change, even though body composition (fat versus lean weight) is changing dramatically. During this period, pay more attention to how your clothing fits than what the scale says.

It's a good idea to have your body composition evaluated, before trying to lose weight, and again period- ically to measure any muscle gain and fat loss from exercise. As I said earlier, your scale weight isn't an accurate indicator of body composition — it can't give you the real picture of the changes you can expect from regular exercise.

Figure 19
Calories Burned Up During 10 Minutes of Continuous Activity

Activity	150#	175#	200#	225#	250#	275#	300#
LOCOMOTION							
Walking – 2 mph	35	40	46	53	58	64	69
One mile – @ 2 mph	105	120	140	157	175	193	210
Walking – 4½ mph	67	78	87	98	110	120	131
One mile – @ 4½ mph	89	103	115	130	147	160	173
Walking Upstairs	175	201	229	259	288	318	350
Walking Downstairs	67	78	88	100	111	122	134
Jogging – 5½ mph	108	127	142	160	178	197	215
Running – 7 mph	141	164	187	208	232	256	280
Running – 12 mph (sprint)	197	230	258	295	326	360	395
Running in place (140 count)	242	284	325	363	405	447	490
Bicycle – 5½ mph	50	58	67	75	83	92	101
Bicycle – 13 mph	107	125	142	160	178	197	216
RECREATION							
Badminton or Volleyball	52	67	75	85	94	104	115
Baseball (except pitcher)	47	54	62	70	78	86	94
Basketball	70	82	93	105	117	128	140
Bowling (nonstop)	67	82	90	100	111	122	133
Canadian Airforce Exercise -0.5 Bx 1A	83	97	108	123	137	152	168
2A	104	122	137	155	173	190	207
3A,4A	147	170	192	217	244	267	290
5A,6A	167	192	217	240	270	300	330
Dancing – moderate	42	49	55	62	69	77	86
Dancing – vigorous	57	67	75	86	94	104	115
Square Dancing	68	80	90	103	113	124	135
Football	83	97	110	123	137	152	167
Golf – foursome	40	47	55	62	68	75	83
Horseback Riding (trot)	67	78	90	102	112	123	134
Ping Pong	38	43	52	58	64	71	78
Skiing – (alpine)	96	113	128	145	160	177	195
Skiing – (cross country)	117	137	158	174	194	214	235
Skiing – (water)	73	92	104	117	130	142	165
Swimming – (backstroke) 20 yd/min	38	43	52	58	64	71	79
Swimming – (breaststroke) 20 yd/min	48	55	63	72	80	88	96
Swimming – crawl 20 yd/min	48	55	63	72	80	88	96
Tennis	67	80	92	103	115	125	135
Wrestling, Judo or Karate	129	150	175	192	213	235	257

Figure 19 (continued)
Calories Burned Up During 10 Minutes of Continuous Activity

Activity	Body Weight						
	150#	175#	200#	225#	250#	275#	300#
PERSONAL ACTIVITIES							
Sleeping	12	14	16	18	20	22	24
Sitting (TV or reading)	12	14	16	18	20	22	24
Sitting (Conversing)	18	21	24	28	30	34	37
Washing/Dressing	32	38	42	47	53	58	63
Standing quietly	14	17	19	21	24	26	28
SEDENTARY OCCUPATION							
Sitting/Writing	18	21	24	28	30	34	37
Light Office Work	30	35	39	45	50	55	60
Standing (Light Activity)	24	28	32	37	40	45	50
HOUSEWORK							
General Housework	41	48	53	60	68	74	81
Washing Windows	42	49	54	61	69	76	83
Making Beds	39	46	52	58	65	75	85
Mopping Floors	46	54	60	68	75	83	91
Light Gardening	36	42	47	53	59	66	73
Weeding Garden	59	69	78	88	98	109	120
Mowing Grass (power)	41	48	53	60	67	74	81
Mowing Grass (manual)	45	53	58	66	74	81	88
Shoveling Snow	78	92	100	117	130	144	160
LIGHT WORK							
Factory Assembly	24	28	32	37	40	45	50
Truck-Auto Repair	42	49	54	61	69	76	83
Carpentry/Farm Work	38	45	51	58	64	71	78
Brick Laying	34	40	45	51	57	62	67
HEAVY WORK							
Chopping Wood	73	86	96	109	121	134	156
Pick & Shovel Work	67	79	88	100	110	120	130

Source: *Habits Not Diets*, by James M. Ferguson, M.D., Bull Publishing Co., 1988. Used with permission.

Chapter 15

Running On Empty
The Dangers of Starvation by Choice

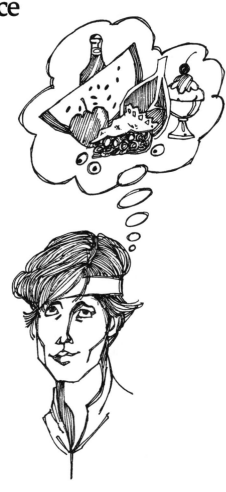

A man who took up cycling became more interested in his overall health and ate less red meat. From there, he decided that fasting would cleanse his body and help him to feel even healthier.

The day before a 200-mile ride he fasted. After 50 miles of the ride he was desperate for food, begging some nourishment from his riding partners. His performance that day was much slower than usual. However, he claimed that fasting "enhanced his experience."

He continued fasting, although his performance kept deteriorating.

Starvation is in. Whether just to try to look like the models or to improve athletic performance, we are prey to a host of misconceptions — from bizarre diet regimens to true eating disorders. They put any athlete at risk — for deterioration in performance, and for serious health consequences.

Low-Carbohydrate Diets

Like so many other people, athletes often search for a "quick" and "easy" way to lose weight. Fad diets are popular because they usually promise the dieter rapid weight loss. The most popular fad diets are usually low in carbohydrate.

The decreased carbohydrate intake causes muscle and liver glycogen depletion. Since water is stored with glycogen, a large amount of water is lost. Dieters cherish this rapid weight (water) loss and assume that it represents fat loss. Actually, their body fat stores are virtually untouched. Eventually, as the body adjusts for the water deficit, the weight loss slows or ceases, and the dieter becomes frustrated and abandons the diet.

Complications associated with low-carbohydrate fad diets include ketosis (increased blood acids), potassium and calcium depletion, dehydration, weakness, nausea, electrolyte loss, gout and possible kidney problems. Vitamin and mineral deficiencies are other potential problems on such unbalanced diets. In addition, low-carbohydrate diets are usually high in fat, and may increase the risk of heart disease when used repeatedly.

Low-carbohydrate fad diets are particularly unsuitable for people who exercise regularly. As you certainly know by now, muscle glycogen is the preferred fuel for endurance exercise, and these diets will reduce muscle glycogen stores. Ketosis also can cause irritability, loss of appetite and nausea — which may further hinder athletic performance. Also, dehydration and electrolyte losses impair temperature regulation and increase the risk of heat illness.

Fasting for Weight Loss

Occasionally even semi-starvation and fasting are used for weight loss. Although well supervised programs such as Optifast can be appropriate for some people, the popular form, relying on popular myth without professional nutrition guidance, can be harmful. Fasting and semi-starvation can cause large losses of water, electrolytes, minerals, glycogen and lean body tissue — and are usually short-lived and thus of questionable value for real fat loss.

What Fad Diets Don't Teach

Fad diets, semi-starvation and fasting are also faulty from a behavioral standpoint, because they tend to reinforce bad eating habits, and distract dieters from the truth that real long-term weight control usually requires fundamental change.

The dieter is not encouraged to learn about the composition, planning and preparation of foods to make well-educated food selections. Rather, most fad diets establish rigid rules and limitations that can be followed only for a short time. Typically, the dieter then abandons the diet and the weight is regained.

Fad diets appeal to the emotions and therefore perpetuate the myth that weight loss can be achieved quickly and easily. Rarely do they address the true need to make basic changes in what are life-long ways of looking at and dealing with food. But the greatest danger associated with these regimens is that the diet will be nutritionally unbalanced and have harmful side effects.

Evaluating Diet Programs

When evaluating a weight loss program, you should consider these points:

1) Does the diet include a variety of foods to ensure nutritional adequacy?

2) Does the program avoid sensational claims such as "magic," "spot reduction," or "eat all you want"?

3) Is the diet's effectiveness well-documented (e.g., the Weight Watchers program) and not based on anecdotal evidence or testimonials?

4) Does it call for behavior and lifestyle changes, and does it incorporate exercise?

5) Does it avoid the use of diuretics and/or appetite suppressants?

Faulty Weight Loss Aids

Diet pills should be avoided entirely. They generally contain a form of stimulant (such as amphetamines), which may suppress the appetite, but only temporarily, so the rate of weight loss (typically one pound per week over the course of several months) tapers off with time. The long-term results are particularly dismaying because the dieters have learned to rely on the pill rather than their own efforts. The lost pounds (and often more) are typically regained, when people stop taking the pills. Also, diet pills containing amphetamines can be addictive, and they can cause insomnia, high blood pressure, headache and dizziness.

Other ineffective "fat-reducers" include vibrating belts, body wraps and electric muscle stimulators. Vibrating belts don't decrease body fat because such passive exercise doesn't increase caloric expenditure — and they have even caused fractures. Body wraps cause temporary water loss from the area that is wrapped, so the person may look thinner for a short time. However, when the water is restored, the figure returns to normal.

Electric muscle stimulators are placed on specific muscle groups and cause them to contract in reaction to a small electric current. They are used for the rehabilitation of injured muscles and do result in increased muscle tone, but they do not increase caloric expenditure enough to result in any body fat loss.

Some people mistakenly believe they can "sweat off fat." (Even professional football players, with professional advice available, talk about losing 10 pounds during a hot training camp workout — it's 95% water.) Exercising with a sweat suit on a warm day and lounging in a sauna will cause weight loss, but it's almost entirely sweat losses. Such loss of body water can be harmful — it can cause dehydration and increased susceptibility to heat illnesses. And of course weight will return to normal when the sweat-induced water loss is replaced.

Energy Efficiency

The metabolism of people who restrict their caloric intake (chronic dieters) and who repeatedly lose and gain weight (yo-yo dieters) may become more efficient in the use of dietary calories. As a result, these individuals may not require as many calories to meet their energy needs as people who have not restricted their caloric intakes. A caloric intake that is considered normal for size, gender, and activity level may cause weight gain for an individual who has continually restricted calories.

What can be done for athletes who have low metabolic rates due to continuous or repeated dieting? They should avoid stringent caloric restrictions, which will reduce their metabolism even more. Gradually adding small amounts of calories (50-100/day) may raise the metabolic rate as long as the athlete keeps exercising. (The increase in metabolic rate is probably due to increased dietary thermogenesis — the energy required for digestion — from the higher caloric intake.) After a while, and over a period of weeks and months, the total caloric intake can then be increased gradually, allowing the metabolic rate to rise accordingly.

The additional calories should be eaten earlier in the day, to help prevent overeating later in the day. The foods added should be predominantly carbohydrate. The rationale for this is two-fold. Athletes need ample carbohydrate to promote glycogen synthesis; and carbohydrate is more likely to be burned for energy than stored as fat.

Eating Disorders

Almost all active people are concerned about their weight. Ideally, this concern will spur them to achieve ideal body composition for health and performance. But with increasing frequency, losing weight becomes an obsession, with the person developing a destructive eating disorder, with distorted views of the need either to avoid any weight gain or to bring about drastic weight loss. Eating disorders, unless recognized and treated, can cause serious physical damage, and even death.

The two eating disorders that are becoming more visible among athletes are *anorexia nervosa* and *bulimia*. Anorexia nervosa is characterized by extreme weight loss, altered body image and an intense fear of becoming obese. Only when they are losing weight do people with anorexia nervosa feel in control of their bodies. They feel an obsessive challenge to continue the weight loss. People with anorexia nervosa consciously deny hunger despite a ravenous appetite, and typically undertake unusually strenuous exercise programs.

The abnormal behavior becomes self-rewarding — as the person loses weight, the sense of control increases. Anorexics typically lose at least 15 to 25% of their body weight and females are usually amenorrheic. But even when people with anorexia nervosa become emaciated, they still think of themselves as fat.

Victims of bulimia — which literally means "ox hunger" — are also overly concerned about their appearance, although they can be under, over or normal weight. They embark on periodic eating binges and then, to preserve their perceived body images, they purge themselves, following the binge with self-induced vomiting, fasting or the use of laxatives or diuretics.

Some people with bulimia will consume between 2,000 and 10,000 calories in just a few hours, then use the purging mechanism to alleviate the shame and guilt of gorging. Bulimic symptoms are seen in about 50% of people with anorexia nervosa.

Family and friends may not be aware of the binge-purge cycle, because people with bulimia are secretive and go to great lengths to conceal all evidence of their actions. Among other health complications, they often develop dental decay, due to the repeated vomiting of highly acidic stomach contents.

Athletes and Weight Loss

Many athletes who engage in sports that require speed and/or vertical motion — like distance running, aquatic diving and gymnastics — feel they would benefit from leaner, lighter bodies. Others, who compete in weight classified sports like wrestling, aspire to make the lowest possible weight class, believing mistakenly, that it will give them a competitive edge. Slimness is also desirable in athletics where the physique is highly visible and artistic style is interpreted through body movement, such as gymnastics, figure skating, dance, and body building.

Some athletes in these sports resort to the tactics of those with eating disorders. When an athlete develops an obsession with food and fatness, it is often difficult to tell whether the obsession is due to the belief that "thin will win," or if there is a true eating disorder.

Both highly motivated exercisers and eating disorder victims share the desire to excel and the desire to control mind and body. Both deny pain, fatigue and hunger. Both experience depression, anxiety, and deprivation when their personal rituals — strenuous exercise and/or dieting — cannot be continued.

People suspected of having an eating disorder should be approached privately by someone they trust. Even if the person is not receptive, he will at least have learned that there is someone to turn to for help in the future. Ideally, the person should be referred to a physician, psychologist or registered dietitian who specializes in treating eating disorders.

Although anyone normally hesitates to talk to a person about a possible eating disorder, ignoring the problem increases the danger to the victim. It is a serious matter. In the most severe cases, people with anorexia nervosa who cannot overcome their aversion to eating eventually become unable to eat, and may actually starve themselves to death.

Complications of both anorexia and bulimia include malnutrition, electrolyte imbalance, dehydration, gastrointestinal problems, heart rhythm irregularities, organ damage, fainting and seizures. Adolescent growth decreases as the disorder continues, potentially leading to permanently stunted growth.

When an eating disorder is detected, ideally an athlete should not be allowed to compete until she or he is under treatment. If the disorder remains untreated, the person may suffer permanent physical injury. Often the person will play down or deny the significance of an injury and keep exercising, thereby causing more damage.

Sources of Help

Many professionals specializing in this area recommend that people who have eating disorders join national eating disorder self-help groups, which provide useful peer support, newsletters and other help. These are non-profit organizations and would appreciate it if requests for information were accompanied by a self-addressed stamped business-size envelope. Among the most popular organizations are:

American Anorexia/Bulimia Association, Inc.
(AABA)
418 East 76th Street
New York, NY 10021
(212) 734-1114

Anorexia Nervosa and Associated Disorders, Inc.
(ANAD)
P.O. Box 7
Highland Park, IL 60035
(708) 831-3438

Anorexia Nervosa and Related Eating Disorders, Inc.
(ANRED)
P.O. Box 5102
Eugene, OR 97405
(503) 344-1144

Bulimia, Anorexia Self-Help
(BASH)
6125 Clayton Avenue, #215
St. Louis, MO 63139
(314) 567-4080

National Anorexic Aid Society, Inc.
(NAAS)
1925 E. Dublin-Granville Road
Columbus, OH 43229
(614) 436-1112

Chapter 16

The Futility of Fads
Don't Buy Into a Miracle Cure

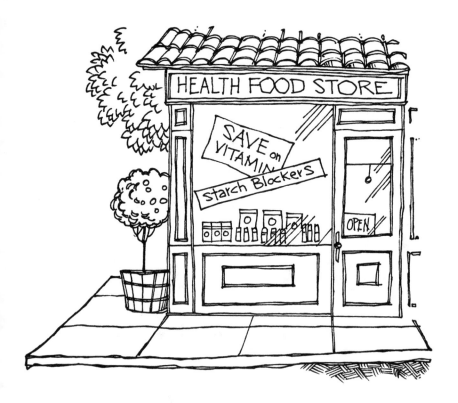

A woman runner was training 70 miles a week for a marathon, which she hoped to finish in two hours and 55 minutes — a goal within her reach.

Her well-meaning coach put her on a juice fast the day before the marathon, thinking it would cleanse her body of wastes and thereby improve her running.

She felt light the morning of the run and ran well for the first quarter of the marathon. As she pushed onto the 13-mile mark though, she felt her strength ebbing. She hit the wall and struggled to finish, relying mainly on her form, which was very good.

She had trained twice as many miles for this marathon, but failed to improve her time. If it hadn't been for her natural ability, she probably wouldn't have even finished.

We want to believe. Even when we've signed up for that magic powder, new wonder diet, new dietary supplement again and again — and been disappointed again and again — we're ready for the next hustle. If we're lucky, it only costs us money, and perhaps some missed trophies.

Faddism

"New endurance performance breakthrough!

"Increases oxygen availability to your muscles.

"Raises your aerobic capacity without additional training.

"Our special product is an oxygen-releasing enzyme extracted from natural foods by a secret process.

"Just send $29.95 for your first 20 capsules."

Sounds too good to be true? It is. We are constantly barraged by advertisements promising that a new wonder product will enhance physical prowess, promote quick weight loss, improve our sex lives, delay aging or restore lost youth, improve our appearance and/or cure our ailments. If you often succumb to these claims, you are a faddist.

A faddist is a person who embraces popular fashions enthusiastically, without demanding any substantial basis. Faddism is successful because we want to believe that there are "magical" alternatives to the standard health practices, sound diet, and hard training that will promote well being and/or improved performance.

Athletes seek that "secret ingredient" which will enhance their workout and give them the edge over their competitors. As a result, they are easy marks for nutritional faddism. And we find a wealth of nutritional supplements which supposedly relieve muscle soreness, boost stamina, speed up healing, increase speed, improve muscle mass and/or reduce body fat.

Often such supplements are recommended by a sincere friend or respected athlete who feels that the product is beneficial. Just as often, the product is endorsed by a food quack.

Food Quacks

Food quacks are fraudulent pretenders who claim to have skills, knowledge or qualifications they do not possess. They can be recognized because they have something to sell. Their motive is your money. Quacks make promises and exaggerated claims. They use an emotional approach. They distrust the health professions and assert that foods needed to meet nutritional needs cannot be purchased in grocery stores. Food quacks exist because food faddists exist.

Most of the time, quacks only do injury to our wallets, promising benefits they can't deliver. But they can do real damage, commonly where necessary medical treatment is delayed at a time when it could be most effective in treating an illness.

Today's nutrition quacks are very adept at mimicking real scientists and health professionals. The quack may have even purchased a Ph.D. from a diploma mill (an unaccredited institution) to appear more credible.

When food quacks assess a person's nutritional status, they use various scientific-appearing "tests" to diagnose nutritional deficiencies and food allergies. They use these tests to appear scientific, convince patients to purchase food supplements, or perhaps to profit directly from the sale of the test itself. The tests used by nutrition quacks include cytotoxic testing, applied kinesiology and hair analysis.

These pseudo-nutritionists use their pseudo-technology to always find something wrong. Their typical "diagnoses" include: food allergies, malabsorption, hypoglycemia, glandular disturbances, adrenal insufficiency, trace vitamin and mineral deficiencies and/or the build-up of various toxins in the body — all scary-sounding problems that are difficult to prove or disprove.

Food quacks often claim they are doing a nutrition assessment, but what constitutes valid nutritional assessment? Nutrition assessment should be part of a general health examination, and when it is it requires the combined expertise of a registered dietitian and a physician. It usually includes a case or medical history, dietary history and clinical evaluations. If neither a registered dietitian or physician is involved, the assessment should be suspect.

Remember that quackery can be very subtle. Fitness oriented people want to believe in something that is mystical or that will improve performance — more than just a prudent diet. In many events where the difference between winning and losing is split seconds, it is not surprising that athletes are susceptible to claims for magical foods and/or nutrients.

The placebo effect by itself can be powerful enough to actually produce benefits: When athletes are convinced that certain foods or supplements improve performance, the belief itself may actually make them perform better, even though there is nothing in the food or supplement that is inherently useful.

Ergogenic Aids

Ergogenic aids represent the trendiest area of sports nutrition. They supposedly enhance performance above levels anticipated under normal conditions. Ergogenic means "work producing." Many athletes believe that ergogenic aids such as amino acids, co-enzyme Q-10, and carnitine will give them a competitive edge. In fact they offer no benefits, and may be harmful.

New ergogenic aids for athletes are constantly emerging. Often these products are marketed without any supportive scientific research to indicate the potential benefits or harmful side effects. Required ingredient lists can be manipulated to support bogus health claims. Some products come and go off the market before studies are done to establish or refute their claims. Prosecutions or other legal actions take years, and the promoter can reap huge benefits during the delay.

If you have questions about a particular supplement, contact a registered dietitian specializing in sports nutrition, or the National Council Against Health Fraud, P.O. Box 1276, Loma Linda, CA, 92354, (714) 824-4690.

True Scientific Advantages

We know that there are definite ways to improve endurance — carbohydrate loading and caffeine ingestion, proper hydration, carbohydrate ingestion during prolonged exercise, and most importantly, a well-balanced diet rich in complex carbohydrates.

There are many factors responsible for performance, and scientific research continues to search out and identify these variables. Valid nutrition concepts are built on such evidence, not rash claims. As researchers continue to investigate fuel usage during exercise, and the effects of food and fluid intake for such exercise, we can continue to improve endurance. To me, that's exciting!

Appendix

Professional Organizations

American College of Sports Medicine (ACSM)
P.0. Box 1440
Indianapolis, IN 46206
(317) 637-9200

Publication: *Medicine and Science in Sports and Exercise*
Purpose: To communicate research on exercise to members and public.
Membership: People in fields of exercise and medicine; 14 categories.

American Dietetic Association Practice Group of Sports and Cardiovascular Nutritionists (SCAN)
216 West Jackson Blvd, Suite 800
Chicago, IL 60606-6995
(312) 899-0040

Publication: *SCAN Pulse*
Purpose: To promote integration of nutrition and exercise
Membership: Dietitians who are members of the American Dietetic Association

Important Journals on Exercise, Nutrition and General Health Promotion

Exercise
American Journal of Sports Medicine
Annals of Sports Medicine
European Journal of Applied Physiology
International Journal of Sports Medicine
Journal of Applied Physiology
Journal of Sports Medicine and Health Physical Fitness
Medicine and Science in Sports and Exercise
Physician and SportsMedicine
Research Quarterly in Exercise and Sport
Sports Medicine

Nutrition
American Journal of Clinical Nutrition
Human Nutrition: Applied
Human Nutrition: Clinical
International Journal of Sports Nutrition
Journal of Nutrition Education
Journal of the American College of Nutrition
Journal of the American Dietetic Association
Nutrition Action
Nutrition Reviews

General Health Promotion
American Journal of Epidemiology
American Journal of Public Health
Annals of Internal Medicine
Clinical Science
Diabetes
Diabetes Care
Federation Proceedings
International Journal of Obesity
Journal of the American Geriatrics Society
Journal of the American Medical Association
Journal of Chronic Diseases
Metabolism
New England Journal of Medicine
Preventive Medicine
Postgraduate Medicine
Psychosomatic Medicine
Smoking and Health Reporter
Western Journal of Medicine

Sample Menus

These sample menus provide examples of diets that generally meet the Dietary Goals for the United States, published by the U.S. Select Committee on Nutrition and Human Needs.

Sample 1,500 Calorie Menu
(Designed to meet U.S. Dietary Goals)

Breakfast

1 cup cream of wheat
2 tablespoons raisins
½ cup orange juice

Lunch

½ whole grain pita bread
⅓ cup seasoned garbanzo beans with lettuce, tomato and onion as filling
½ cup cooked broccoli
½ mango
1 cup low-fat milk

Dinner

4 ounces lean beef
1 baked potato with
2 teaspoons margarine
½ cup spinach salad
1 tablespoon French dressing
Yogurt shake:
   1 cup low-fat yogurt
   ½ banana
   ¾ cup strawberries

Approximately: 56% Carbohydrate; 17% Protein; 27% Fat.

Sample 2,000 Calorie Menu
(Designed to meet U.S. Dietary Goals)

Breakfast
⅓ cup bran cereal
1 cup low-fat milk
1 banana
1 piece raisin toast
½ cup grapefruit juice

Lunch
Tuna Melt (Use Pam or equivalent
   to grill)
   2 slices whole wheat bread
   3 ounces tuna mixed with 1
      teaspoon mayonnaise, celery
      and green onion, chopped
      and folded in
   1 ounce Cheddar cheese
   tomato slice
carrot and celery sticks
1 cup apple juice
1 cup low-fat yogurt with
1 cup raspberries

Dinner
Stir fry in 2 teaspoons oil:
   4 ounces chicken, no skin
   1½ cup vegetables
1½ cups brown rice
1 orange

Snack
1 cup low-fat milk
1 blueberry muffin

Approximately: 57% Carbohydrate; 14% Protein; 29% Fat.

U.S. Recommended Dietary Allowances

MINERALS

Adult U.S.RDA Female/Male	Functions	Sources
Calcium 800 mg	Bone formation, enzyme reactions, muscle contractions	Dairy products, green leafy vegetables, beans
Iron 15/10 mg	Hemoglobin formation, muscle growth and function, energy production	Lean meat, beans, dried fruit, some green leafy vegetables
Magnesium 280/350 mg	Energy production, muscle relaxation, nerve conduction	Grains, nuts, meats, beans
Sodium EMR* 500 mg	Nerve impulses, muscle action, body fluid balance	Table salt, small amounts in most food except fruit
Potassium EMR* 2000 mg	Fluid balance, muscle action, glycogen and protein synthesis	Bananas, orange juice, fruits, vegetables
Zinc 12/15 mg	Tissue growth and healing, immunity, gonadal development	Meat, shellfish, oysters grains
Copper ESI* 1.5-3 mg	Hemoglobin formation, energy production, immunity	Whole grains, beans, nuts dried fruit, shellfish
Selenium 55/70 mcg	Anti-oxidant, protects against free radicals, enhances vitamin E	Meat, seafood, grains
Chrominum ESI* 50-200 mcg	Part of glucose tolerance factor — helps insulin	Whole grains, meat, cheese, beer
Manganese ESI* 2-5 mg	Bone and tissue development, fat synthesis	Nuts, grains, beans, tea, fruits, vegetables
Iodine 150 mg	Regulates metabolism	Iodized salt, seafood
Flouride 1.5-4 mg	Formation of bones and tooth enamel	Tap water, tea, coffee, rice, spinach, lettuce
Phosphorus 800 mg	Builds bones and teeth, metabolism	Meat, fish, dairy products, carbonated drinks

EMR — estimated minimum requirement
ESI — estimated safe and adequate dietary intake

U.S. Recommended Dietary Allowances

VITAMINS

Adult U.S.RDA Female/Male	Functions	Sources
Vitamin C 60 mg	Collagen formation, immunity, anti-oxidant	Citrus fruits, tomatoes, strawberries, potatoes, broccoli, cabbage
Vitamin B_1 (Thiamin) 1.1/1.5 mg	*Energy production, central* nervous system	*Meat, whole grain cereals,* milk, beans
Niacin 15-19 mg	Energy production, synthesis of fat and amino acids	Peanut butter, whole grain cereals, greens, meat, poultry, fish
Vitamin B_6 (Pyridoxine) 1.6/2.0 mg	Protein metabolism, hemoglobin synthesis, energy production	Whole grain cereals, bananas, meat, spinach, cabbage, Lima beans
Folacin 180/200 mcg	New cell growth, red blood cell production	Greens, mushrooms, liver
Vitamin B_{12} (Cobalmin) 2 mcg	Energy metabolism, red blood cell production, central nervous system	Animal foods
Vitamin A 800/1,000 mcg	Vision, skin, anti-oxidant, immunity	Milk, egg yolk, liver, yogurt, carrots, greens
Vitamin D 5 mcg	Formation of bones, aids absorption of calcium	Sunlight, fortified dairy products, eggs, fish
Vitamin E 8/10 mg	Anti-oxidant, protects unsaturated fats in cells from damage	Vegetable oils, margarines grains
Vitamin K 65-80 mcg	Blood clotting	Greens, liver

Index